CONTEMPORARY PATTERNS
OF BREAST-FEEDING

The World Health Organization is a specialized agency of the United Nations with primary responsibility for international health matters and public health. Through this organization, which was created in 1948, the health professions of more than 150 countries exchange their knowledge and experience with the aim of making possible the attainment by all citizens of the world by the year 2000 of a level of health that will permit them to lead a socially and economically productive life.

By means of direct technical cooperation with its Member States, and by stimulating such cooperation among them. WHO promotes the development of comprehensive health services, the prevention and control of diseases, the improvement of environmental conditions, the development of health manpower, the coordination and development of biomedical and health services research, and the planning and implementation of health programmes.

These broad fields of endeavour encompass a wide variety of activities, such as developing systems of primary health care that reach the whole population of Member countries; promoting the health of mothers and children: combating malnutrition: controlling malaria and other communicable diseases including tuberculosis and leprosy; having achieved the eradication of smallpox, promoting mass immunization campaigns against a number of other preventable diseases; improving mental health; providing safe water supplies; and training health personnel of all categories.

Progress towards better health throughout the world also demands international cooperation in such matters as establishing international standards for biological substances, pesticides and pharmaceuticals; formulating environmental health criteria; recommending international nonproprietary names for drugs; administering the International Health Regulations; revising the International Classification of Diseases, Injuries, and Causes of Death; and collecting and disseminating health statistical information.

Further information on many aspects of WHO's work is presented in the Organization's publications.

CONTEMPORARY PATTERNS OF BREAST-FEEDING

Report on the WHO Collaborative Study on Breast-feeding

WORLD HEALTH ORGANIZATION
GENEVA
1981

ISBN 92 4 156067 3

The designations employed and the presentation of the material in this publication do not imply the expression of any opinion whatsoever on the part of the Secretariat of the World Health Organization concerning the legal status of any country, territory, city or area or of its authorities, or concerning the delimitation of its frontiers or boundaries.

The mention of specific companies or of certain manufacturers' products does not imply that they are endorsed or recommended by the World Health Organization in preference to others of a similar nature that are not mentioned. Errors and omissions excepted, the names of proprietary products are distinguished by initial capital letters.

TYPESET IN INDIA
PRINTED IN SWITZERLAND

80/4840 – Macmillan/Atar – 12000

Contents

Preface

In recent years the importance of breast-feeding as a basis for healthy child growth and development has become increasingly recognized. As scientific evidence accumulates on the unique nutritional and immunological properties of breast-milk, as well as on the effects of breast-feeding on reproductive function and mother–child bonding, concern is increasing about the possible effects of a decline in breast-feeding on the well-being of children, especially in the Third World.

The success both of national and of international programmes to promote better feeding of infants and young children, especially breast-feeding, depends on adequate information on contemporary patterns of infant feeding among different socioeconomic and cultural groups. It was with this intention that the WHO Collaborative Study on Breast-feeding, reported here, was developed.

The first phase, dealing in particular with the prevalence and duration of breast-feeding, was conducted in nine countries, seven of them in the Third World. A second phase, dealing with the volume and composition of breast-milk in relation to maternal health and socioeconomic characteristics, is now under way.

The results from the first phase are already serving as a basis for planning and carrying out action programmes in the nine countries that were surveyed and in other parts of the world as well. They are also being used in developing national programmes of education, training, and public information designed to alert different social groups to the need for more attention to this important subject.

Acknowledgements

The World Health Organization wishes to express its special thanks to the Principal Investigators listed below, whose untiring efforts made this study possible. A great debt of gratitude is owed also to the Consultants for their invaluable advice and assistance. In particular, the Organization wishes to acknowledge the guidance and support so willingly given by the late Dr Nathalie Masse and the late Professor Bo Vahlquist. Their concern for children and for the development of scientific approaches to infant feeding was a motivating force in the progression of this study, and it is to them that this report is dedicated.

Thanks are also due to the collaborating centres and national teams in the nine participating countries and to the 23 000 mothers who, together with their families, took part in the study.

The study was developed in close collaboration with the International Children's Centre, Paris, and was carried out with the generous financial support of the United Nations Fund for Population Activities and the Swedish International Development Authority.

Participants in the WHO Collaborative Study on Breast-feeding: First phase

Principal investigators and national teams

Chile

Dr A. Patri, Centre for Nutrition, Growth, and Development, University of Chile, Santiago

R. Anderson, V. Celis, E. Diaz, E. Fernández, M. Fernández, M. González, H. Jara, G. Jiménez, J. Ugarte, J. Valenzuela

Ethiopia

Dr Z. Gebriel, Ethiopian Nutrition Institute, Addis Ababa S. Bekele, A. Teshome Demeke, M. Wolde Georgis, F. Ketsela, A. Mario Maffi, A. Haile Mariam, A. Gebre Yohannes

Guatemala

Dr J. J. Urrutia, Institute of Nutrition for Central America and Panama (INCAP), Guatemala

B. Garcia

Hungary

Dr I. Öry, Department of Mother, Child, and Youth Care, Ministry of Health, Budapest

P. Cholnoky, R. Agfalvy, A. Klinger, A. Pinter, G. Talas

India

Dr B. Belavady, National Institute of Nutrition, Hyderabad

B. V. S. Thimmayama, K. Visweswara Rao, M. Vidyavathi, A. P. Likhite,

A. F. Zaidi, R. I. Devi, K. S. Nargis, N. Khatri, P. Harinath, L. S. Monica, G. J. Ratnakumari, S. Vasir, S. Fatima

Nigeria

Dr A. Omololu, Department of Human Nutrition, University of Ibadan, Ibadan

S. O. Oparinde, E, Adeyi

Philippines

Dr V. B. Guzman, Department of Community Health, Institute of Public Health, University of the Philippines, Manila

A. Villanueva, L. V. del Castillo, T. R. Lariosa, N. Aquino, J. Regio, A. del Rosario, J. A. Palad, P. Ramos, C. Villas, S. Pamatian, T. Tan, D. Lara, M. Reyes

Sweden

*Dr Y. Hofvander, Department of Paediatrics, University Hospital, Uppsala

C. Hillervik, E. Kylberg

Zaire

*Dr H. L. Vis, Institute of Scientific Research, Kinshasa; Department of Paediatrics, Université libre de Bruxelles, Belgium

M. Demaegd, P. Hennart, M. Ruchababisha-Migabo

Marketing study

*Dr B. Wickström, Department of Business Administration, University of Gothenburg, Sweden

Consultants

Mr W. Z. Billewicz, Medical Research Council, Reproduction and Growth Unit, Newcastle-upon-Tyne, England

The late Dr N. Masse, International Children's Centre, Paris, France

Dr M. Péchevis, International Children's Centre, Paris, France

Dr A. M. Thomson, Medical Research Council, Reproduction and Growth Unit, Newcastle upon Tyne, England

The late Dr B. Vahlquist, University Hospital, Uppsala, Sweden

WHO Secretariat

Dr M. Behar, Nutrition, Division of Family Health

Dr M. Carballo, Maternal and Child Health, Division of Family Health (*Study Coordinator*)

Dr E. DeMaeyer, Nutrition, Division of Family Health

Mr P. C. Kaufmann, Health Statistical Methodology, Division of Health Statistics

Dr A. Petros-Barvazian, Division of Family Health

Mrs E. Royston, Division of Family Health

Dr G. Sterky, Maternal and Child Health, Division of Family Health

---

*Also acted as a consultant to the study.

1. Introduction

The late Professor Bo Vahlquist was a key proponent of breast-feeding and, as a scientist and paediatrician, devoted much of his time to reviving interest in this important aspect of child care.

His encouragement and support contributed significantly to the development of the WHO Collaborative Study on Breast-feeding and he was an invaluable source of guidance throughout the first phase. Because of his interest in and knowledge of the subject, Professor Vahlquist was asked to prepare the introduction to this report. This was condensed and edited after his untimely death.

In all mammalian species the reproductive cycle comprises both pregnancy and breast-feeding; in the absence of the latter, none of those species, man included, could have survived.

While it is difficult to state with any degree of accuracy what is the worldwide proportion of mothers who cannot breast-feed, it is unlikely to exceed 10%. Historical data and what is known of the situation today in rural areas of non-industrialized countries would appear to support this view. There is no reason to believe that any significant change has taken place in the biology of the contemporary woman that would make her less able to lactate and breast-feed than her predecessors of a few generations ago.

There are, of course, certain factors that can have an unfavourable influence on breast-feeding, in particular the health and nutritional status of the mother. Experience has shown, however, that mothers with nutritional deficiencies can, and often do, produce amounts of milk that are only slightly less than average. More importantly, their milk does not vary significantly in composition from that of other mothers and can thus make a vital contribution to infant health and well-being.

One aspect, however, seems to have varied considerably over the last half century or so and from one cultural milieu to another: the duration of breast-feeding and the point at which additional foods are introduced. For, while the infant requires very little food other than breast-milk during the first 4–6 months, it has become quite common in some parts of the world to introduce supplements much earlier.

In the early part of this century, semi-solid and solid supplements such as purées of fruit, vegetables, eggs, meat, and fish were generally recommended for infants of about 12 months, and quite a stir was created in 1921 when Jundell presented evidence that infants would accept, tolerate, and benefit from supplements introduced from the age of 6 months (*15*). With time, it even became common for the health professions to recommend supplements from the age of 3 months with the purpose of adapting the child "in good time" to new taste and texture experiences. The development of industrially produced alternatives to home-based supplements also no doubt played a role in the phenomenon of the earlier introduction of solids and semi-solids; they were readymade, convenient, and often recommended by health workers.

As the idea of early supplementation became more accepted, however, it became increasingly apparent that many mothers were introducing other foods considerably earlier than the third month, and this practice was rightly criticized as not only unnecessary, but indeed physiologically inappropriate (*4*, *17*).

Because of growing concern about this practice, statements were issued by a number of bodies to the effect that, given a favourable environment, the appropriate time for the introduction of supplementary foods was around 4 months post partum (*9*, *27*).

This, of course, is not to say that until then all biological mothers had breast-fed their infants fully for over 6 months, for indeed there have always been alternatives. Since time immemorial, for instance, wet-nursing, or the practice of breast-feeding by someone other than the mother, has been used when for one reason or another the child would have otherwise been deprived of human milk. The tradition of wet-nursing depended upon the availability of women willing and able to provide this service and of a social system that supported and encouraged the practice. In Greek and Roman society and later in mediaeval Europe, recourse to wet-nurses became relatively popular among economically advantaged women. It permitted them to have fewer responsibilities and at the same time ensured that their infants would benefit from "rich milk from a robust and harmonious servant" (*8*, *29*).

It was widely believed that a new biological bond was created between the infant and the wet-nurse. In some cases, it was even held that marriage between the wet-nurse's own child and any other she had breast-fed would be incestuous. Not only was the wet-nurse seen as a source of nourishment for the child, but it was felt that her mental and emotional characteristics would be passed on to the sucking child. Emphasis was placed on the need to select wet-nurses carefully, with due consideration to their background; in France, Germany and Sweden for example, special agencies came into being to help check the health and social credentials of wet-nurses.

Such was the importance attached to wet-nursing that in Rosen von Rosenstein's textbook of 1764 (*26*) no fewer than 14 pages were "On nurses". Almost 150 years later, von Pfaundler & Schlossmann's *Handbuch der Kinderheilkunde* (*21*) still contained five pages on the subject.

But as economic situations changed and job opportunities for women improved, the popularity of wet-nursing as an occupation decreased, even though many paediatric departments continued to employ wet-nurses; in the 1940s, for example, many clinics in Sweden still made budgetary provision for them. In many traditional societies, the importance of wet-nursing is still recognized, and the fact that in these societies the extended family has been maintained more effectively has no doubt helped support the practice.

As interest in wet-nursing decreased, new knowledge about the preservation of human milk made other alternatives possible. In 1910, for example, the first milk bank was established in Boston, USA. Using deep-freezing techniques that permitted milk to be kept sterile over a period of months with little change except in taste, a large number of such banks soon opened throughout North America and Europe. Such was the turnover of milk in these banks that special organizations were needed for the health assessment of the mothers using them and for the collection and quality control of the milk. It was not until infant-feeding formulas became more sophisticated that interest in milk banks gradually decreased.

Interestingly enough, although the domestication of cattle goes back 10 000 years in some areas of the world, animal milks were, with few exceptions, not perceived as an alternative to mother's milk until relatively recently. In the second half of the eighteenth century, Rosen Von Rosenstein (*26*), Armstrong (*1*), and Underwood (*27*) all referred to the modification of animal milk so as to meet the young infant's particular needs, but on the whole they were pessimistic about the effects of the early introduction of anything other than mother's milk.

In the 1880s cow's milk began to be used as a source of supplementary food in the innovative child welfare clinics that had been set up in France to enable children to have regular health checks, including weighing. While these centres strongly encouraged breast-feeding, they also provided sterilized cow's milk, sometimes with cream and sugar added, free of charge to children felt to be in special need. In time, similar clinics and practices became more widespread in other European countries, but by the 1920s interest in the "*gouttes de lait*", as they were called, began to dwindle in Sweden and elsewhere and in general the provision of cow's milk through child health centres appears to have had little effect on breast-feeding practices.

The late nineteenth century saw the first systematic endeavours in the field of artificial feeding, which led to carefully calculated mixtures mainly involving water, sugar, and flour and gradually modified to suit children of different ages. The resulting "formulas", while crude in comparison with the sophisticated products available today, nevertheless represented a considerable improvement over many of the paps that were current at the time and prepared with little regard to digestibility. Budin in France, Biedert and Heubner in Germany, and Meigs and Rotch in the USA were among the most notable pioneers in this field. Thus, in the USA, where Meigs popularized the scientific basis for modifying cow's milk so as to provide a digestible formula for infants, the foundation had been laid by the turn of the century for the systematic feeding of infants using milks other than human milk.

With Pasteur's discovery of the fermentation process and the ensuing explosion of new knowledge in the microbiological field came a revolution in the understanding of food hygiene and preparation, coinciding with improvements in sanitation, water, and other facilities for food preservation.

Nevertheless infant feeding, even using animal milk, continued to be essentially a home-based process until the late 1920s, when the food industry began to prepare first "half products" and then "complete" formulas. By the latter part of the 1930s, the preparation of formulas had moved from the kitchen to the factory, the result being an increasingly sophisticated and specialized range of products designed to meet all the individual food requirements of infants and young children at different ages.

Initially developed in industrialized countries to meet a specific need, breast-milk substitutes gradually became more widespread and are now commonplace in many parts of the Third World. Their introduction into the developing countries is often associated with a whole series of problems: poor environmental sanitation and water supply, as well as inadequate facilities for the proper cleaning of bottles and teats, combined with an economic situation in which the cost of formulas is often prohibitive and their over-dilution frequent. Their wide, often indiscriminate availability is considered by many observers to contribute to the decline of breast-feeding in those countries.

Variations in patterns of breast-feeding were already discernible by the end of the 19th century; Knodel & van de Walle (*16*) suggest, for example, that in central Europe and especially in parts of Germany there were considerable changes in the frequency and duration of breast-feeding at that period.

In the USA, where in 1922 Woodbury (*30*) calculated that about 90% of babies were being breast-fed at 12 months, the 1920s and 1930s also saw the beginning of a decline in the practice. This became even more pronounced in the 1950s, and Meyer (*19*) reports that the prevalence of breast-feeding on discharge from hospital fell from 38% in 1946 to 21% in 1956 and to 18% in 1966. Fomon (*10*), however, suggests that by the early 1970s there was a slight upward trend and that in 1974 about 15% of all babies 4 months of age were being breast-fed.

The trend observed in the USA was followed, although about 15–20 years later, in a number of European countries; in eastern Europe it appeared later still. A variety of factors was probably involved, including the availability of breast-milk substitutes and their marketing, as well as changes in the role of women in society, in hospital practices especially with respect to the delivery and care of the newborn, and in attitudes of health personnel to the preparation of mothers for breast-feeding.

The effects on infant health of these changing patterns of feeding were recorded by a number of people. Böckh, one of the earliest observers, studied infant mortality in Berlin during three one-year periods at intervals of 10 years (1885–86, 1895–96 and 1905–06) and, relating the findings to feeding patterns, observed that mortality under one year of age was much higher among artifically fed infants (*6*).

Similarly, in Britain at the beginning of the century Howarth (*12*), in a study covering more than 8000 children in Derby, reported that mortality was three times higher among the babies who had been "hand-fed" from an early age than among the breast-fed babies.

In the USA, some fifteen years later, Woodbury (*30*) observed that, among more than 22 000 infants from eight cities, mainly located in eastern states, mortality figures were 3–6 times higher for those who were artificially fed; mortality rates for infants aged up to 9 months were almost five times as high among those artificially fed as among those who were breast-fed. The same trend emerged from the studies of Grulee et al. (*11*) who, using data on 20 000 infants in Chicago between 1924 and 1929, showed that mortality was 10 times higher among those who were artificially fed; this figure was particularly striking since the children included in the study were all under monthly supervision at health centres. Mannheimer (*18*), analysing infant mortality figures from Stockholm, found that, even as late as the 1940s, the mortality risk for artificially fed infants was 2–3 times that for breast-fed infants, a fact that was as true for upper-income groups as for others.

It must be noted, however, especially with respect to the earlier studies quoted, that the foods that were used as substitutes for mother's milk were often nutritionally unsatisfactory, while the conditions of hygiene and general care in which they were used were often grossly poor and simply increased the normal risks to which the early weaned baby was exposed. From the 1940s onwards, reports from industrialized countries increasingly suggested that mortality rates for both early and late weaned infants did not differ widely, provided that the infants were under good health supervision.

In other parts of the world, however, the situation has remained much the same and, for the large groups below the poverty line in non-industrialized countries, the excess mortality related to early weaning of infants continues to be high (*22*, *25*). Some authors (*3*, *20*) have nevertheless felt that, in Third World countries too, infant mortality has tended to decline at the same time as breast-feeding has declined, going so far as to suggest that early artificial feeding might actually have had a favourable effect.

Of course, one could just as well say that, in spite of the progressively earlier introduction of artificial feeding, other factors—for example, improved standards of living, sanitation, and access to health services—have had a positive effect on infant health. When, following the Second World War, European countries began to experience a serious decline in breast-feeding, infant mortality rates in those countries had already generally fallen below 50 per 1000—in Sweden, even below 20 per 1000. Under these conditions, the progressively earlier introduction of artificial feeding obviously did not have much influence on the continued fall in infant mortality. But this was a very different situation from that prevailing today in the poverty-stricken areas of the Third World and elsewhere.

As knowledge on the relationship between health and the feeding of infants and young children accumulated, so did interest in the possible revival of breast-feeding. Whereas, up to the 1960s, it had been relatively widely held that the decline in breast-feeding was a "fact of modern life", this premise began to be increasingly questioned and it was wondered whether the trend was really irreversible. A series of arguments in favour of breast-feeding emerged, the main points of which are as follows.

1. Artificial feeding from an early age represents the "world's largest experiment without controls" (concerned not so much with the short-range as the potential long-range effects—atherosclerosis, hypertension, obesity, allergy to non-specific proteins, etc.).

2. While not excluding it, artificial feeding from an early age cannot guarantee the skin-to-skin contact between mother and breast-fed child that helps create the bond between them.

3. It has become strikingly evident that even the most sophisticated and carefully adapted formulas can never replicate human milk. In addition to species-specific differences in protein composition, it is now evident that human milk has anti-infective properties, implying that it is a "live" fluid in a way that cannot be mimicked in an artificial formula.

4. When income is low and education poor, the superiority of breast-feeding becomes even more marked, and breast-feeding may in fact represent the only way, in such a context, of really giving a child a fair chance of survival.

5. Breast-feeding has a vital child-spacing effect which is especially important in Third World countries where the availability or acceptability of modern family planning methods may be limited.

As interest in the subject increased, so did the number of reports of the decline of breast-feeding in different parts of the Third World. Unfortunately many of these tended to be more anecdotal than scientifically based and, while they no doubt represented real situations as perceived by observers, they were not of a sufficiently factual kind to stimulate action at the international level. Such scientific studies as were available, moreover, were often based on small and selective population groups or were not methodologically similar, thus making comparative analyses difficult.

This, of course, did not prevent efforts being made to promote breast-feeding or appeals to various organizations and groups to provide the type of support needed to reactivate the practice. In 1956, for example, La Leche League International was formed in the USA, going on to produce a number of books, pamphlets, and periodicals aimed at the promotion and management of breast-feeding and, in fact, arousing considerable interest in the subject. While its effects may not be easily recognizable from national statistics, La Leche League was undoubtedly of vital assistance in "keeping the pot boiling"; more recently, it has encouraged the formation of similar groups of mothers in a number of other countries. Today such groups advise, assist and encourage newly delivered mothers on matters related to breast-feeding and act on an individual basis in more than 40 countries.

During the 1970s, the aims and work of groups such as these were reinforced by the emergence in many societies of progressively stronger "back to nature" movements, in whose philosophy of a more natural life-style breast-feeding in the traditional way was given an important place. Feminist groups, moreover, had no objection to the presentation of breast-feeding as a normal and important part of the reproductive cycle.

At the level of the international agencies interest was also growing. The Protein-Calorie Advisory Group (PAG) of the United Nations System, an important advisory body from 1956 to 1977, established a number of *ad hoc* groups, one of which, initiated in 1969, dealt with the question of feeding the pre-school child and presented a document containing a section on the sociocultural dynamics of breast-feeding (*23*). A passage from this section is worth quoting here:

> A cornerstone of any public health nutrition programme for the prevention of childhood malnutrition must be the need to promote an optimal lactation pattern in the community.

Gradually PAG became more involved in other aspects of breast-feeding, with particular reference to the countries of the Third World. Since one of the factors contributing to the decline in breast-feeding, particularly in urban areas, was undoubtedly the inappropriate promotion of breast-milk substitutes by the baby-food industry, the PAG arranged a series of conferences on the topic, inviting paediatricians, industrial representatives, and representatives of pertinent United Nations bodies to take part (Bogotá, 1970; Paris, 1972; New York, 1973; Singapore, 1974). The last of these conferences led to important revisions in the group's "Recommendations on policies and practices in infant and young child feeding" (*24*).

In May 1974, the Twenty-seventh World Health Assembly also took a clear stand on breast-feeding. Its resolution WHA27.43 on this issue

> URGES Member countries to review sales promotion activities on baby foods and to introduce appropriate remedial measures, including advertisement codes and legislation where necessary,

showing a concern similar to that expressed the same year by the World Food Conference in its Resolution .V, which included the following recommendation:

> That governments consider the key role of women and take steps to improve their nutrition, their educational levels and their working conditions; and . . . encourage them and enable them to breastfeed their children.

In the same way, a number of other specialized agencies of the United Nations, such as UNICEF, FAO and ILO, have indicated their interest in programmes for the promotion of breast-feeding, either as separate ventures or as integral parts of maternal and child health and primary health care activities.

Among nongovernmental groups, the International Paediatric Association (IPA) has dealt with breast-feeding promotion in its recommendations (*13*) on "New urban families" (the subject of a workshop held during its international congress in Vienna in 1971). The Association later went on to propose a series of recommendations for programmes to encourage breast-feeding (*14*). These dealt with a variety of subjects, including the need for better training of health personnel and for better information to mothers, policy-makers, etc., as well as measures to eliminate the worst excesses of the commercial exploitation of artificial infant-feeding formulas. The following paragraphs from the proceedings of the Montreux conference (*14*) deserve quotation:

> Sales promotion activities of organizations marketing baby milks and feeding bottles, that run counter to the general intent expressed in this document, must be curtailed by every means available to the profession, including, where necessary and feasible, legislation to control unethical practice.
>
> Dissemination of propaganda about artificial feeding and distribution of samples of artificial baby foods in maternity units should be banned immediately.

Both the International Union of Nutritional Sciences (IUNS) and the International Planned Parenthood Federation (IPPF), through its Commission No. III (Human development, with special reference to the mother and child), have taken an active part in discussions on the promotion of breast-feeding and jointly convened a working party on lactation, fertility and the working woman (Bellagio, July 1977).

Reference should also be made to the Swedish standards for the marketing of infant foods worked out by a group of paediatricians in 1964 (*2*), which proposed markedly innovative strategies for regulatory action to safeguard breast-feeding.

It was in Vienna in 1971, on the occasion of the Thirteenth International Paediatric Congress, that the desirability of a multinational study on breast-feeding was advanced and the following year, under the auspices of the International Children's Centre, a colloquium on the subject was held in Abidjan (*7*). The participants were unanimous in their view that traditional breast-feeding patterns were being eroded in many areas of the Third World and that measures to stop and, if possible, reverse this trend were desperately needed. It was also agreed that WHO should play a leading part in that connexion, working in close contact with the International Children's Centre. It was recommended that the study should be carried out in two phases, the first dealing with the prevalence and duration of breast-feeding, and the second with the volume and composition of breast-milk.

Both phases, however, have the same objective, namely to lay the ground for meaningful *action programmes* adapted to national needs. For, if feeding practices (and, with them, the health and welfare of children) are to be improved, it will be through the application of scientific findings and the modification, where necessary, of those practices and routines that have developed at the family, health service, and community levels.

There is no reason to accept the premise that breast-feeding is incompatible with modern industrialized society, and every reason to believe that, with adequate social sensitivity to the needs of mothers and children and with appropriate supportive measures to help meet those needs, breast-feeding can retain its integral place in the process of human reproduction and child development.

For the vulnerable infant and young child, an effective public effort to counter the current trend [decline in breast-feeding in low-income countries] may be of greater significance than any other form of nutrition intervention (*5*).

It is with this consideration in mind that WHO has undertaken the current collaborative study.

REFERENCES

1. ARMSTRONG, G. *An essay on the diseases most fatal to infants*, London, T. Cadell, 1767.
2. A Swedish code of ethics for marketing of infant foods (1977) *Acta paediatrica scandinavica,* **66**: 129–132 (1977)
3. AYKROYD, W. R. Is breast feeding best for all infants, everywhere? *Nutrition today,* **12**: 15–18 (1977).
4. BEAL, V. On the acceptance of solid foods, and other food patterns, of infants and children. *Pediatrics,* **20**: 448–456 (1957).
5. BERG, A. *The nutrition factor*, Washington, DC, Brookings Institution, 1976, p. 106.
6. BÖCKH, R. Bericht, betreffend die Sterblichkeit der Kinder nach der Ernährungsweise. In: *Internationalen Kongress für Hygiene und Demographie*, Vienna, 1887 (and later papers).
7. CENTRE INTERNATIONAL DE L'ENFANCE. *Colloque sur l'allaitement maternel, Abidjan, 14–16 novembre 1972.* Paris, Centre International de l'Enfance, 1973.
8. DAVIDSON, W. D. & DURHAM, N. C. A brief history of infant feeding. *Journal of pediatrics,* **43**: 74–87 (1953).
9. EUROPEAN SOCIETY FOR PAEDIATRIC GASTROENTEROLOGY AND NUTRITION, COMMITTEE ON NUTRITION. Guidelines on infant nutrition. I. Recommendations for the composition of an adapted formula *Acta paediatrica scandinavica, Suppl.,* **262**: 1–20 (1977).
10. FOMON, S. J. *Infant nutrition*, 2nd ed. Philadelphia, London, and Toronto, Saunders, 1974.
11. GRULEE, G. G., HEYWORTH, N. S. & HERRON, P. H. Breast and artificial feeding. Influence on morbidity and mortality of twenty thousand infants. *Journal of the American Medical Association,* **103**: 735–738 (1934).
12. HOWARTH, W. J. The influence of feeding on the mortality of infants. *Lancet,* **2**: 210–213 (1905).
13. INTERNATIONAL PAEDIATRIC ASSOCIATION. New urban families. *Acta paediatrica scandinavica,* **61**: 226–229 (1972); *Australian pediatric journal, Suppl.,* **2**: 45–47 (1973).
14. INTERNATIONAL PAEDIATRIC ASSOCIATION. Recommendations for action programs to encourage breast feeding. *IPA bulletin,* **4**: 19–22 (1975).
15. JUNDELL, I. On mixed diet during the first year of life. *Acta paediatrica,* **1**: 240–255 (1921–22).
16. KNODEL, J. & VAN DE WALLE, E. Breast feeding, fertility and infant mortality: an analysis of some early German data. *Population studies,* **21**: 109–131 (1967).
17. MCKEITH, R. & WOOD, C. *Infant feeding and feeding practices*, 4th ed. London, Churchill, 1971.
18. MANNHEIMER, E. Mortality of breast fed and bottle fed infants – a comparative study. *Acta genetica,* **5**: 134–163 (1954).

19. MEYER, H. F. Breastfeeding in the United States: extent and possible trend. *Pediatrics*, **22**: 116–121 (1958)
20. MULLER, H. R. *Nutrition and infant mortality*, 1975 (paper presented at court proceedings in Berne), pp. 9–20.
21. PFAUNDLER, M. VON & SCHLOSSMANN, A. *Handbuch der Kinderheilkunde*, 2nd ed. Leipzig, F. C. W. Vogel, 1910–1912 vol. 1, pp. 156–180
22. PLANK, S. J. & MILANESI, M. L. Infant feeding and infant mortality in rural Chile. *Bulletin of the World Health Organization*, **48**: 203–210 (1973).
23. PROTEIN-CALORIE ADVISORY GROUP. Feeding the preschool child (FAO/WHO/UNICEF document 1.14/5:1–16), 1971.
24. PROTEIN-CALORIE ADVISORY GROUP. Recommendations on policies and practices in infant and young child feeding and proposals for action to implement them. *PAG bulletin*, **5**:1–4 (1975).
25. PUFFER, R. R. & SERRANO, C. V. *Patterns of mortality in childhood*. Washington, DC, Pan American Health Organization, 1973, pp. 257–271.
26. ROSEN VON ROSENSTEIN, N. *Underrättelser om Barn-Sjukdomar och deras Bote-Medel. Tilförene styckewis utgifne uti de sma Almanachorna, nu samlade, tilökte och förbättrade.* Stockholm, Lars Salvius, 1764 (English edition: *The diseases of children and their remedies*. London, T. Cadell, 1776).
27. UNDERWOOD, M. *A treatise on the diseases of children with general directions for the management of infants from the birth; adapted to domestic use*. London, J. Mathews, 1797.
28. UNITED KINGDOM. HEALTH AND SOCIAL SUBJECTS. *Present-day practice in infant feeding. Report of a working party of the panel on child nutrition, Committee on medical aspects of food policy*. London, Her Majesty's Stationery Office, 1974.
29. WICKES, I.G. A history of infant feeding. *Archives of disease in childhood*, **28**: 151–158, 232–240, 332–340, 416–422, 495–502 (1953).
30. WOODBURY, R. M. The relation between breast and artificial feeding and infant mortality. *American journal of hygiene*, **2**: 668–687 (1922).

2. Design of the study

The first phase of the Collaborative Study on Breast-feeding consists of (*a*) the basic study, involving interviews with mothers, and (*b*) complementary surveys using background data collected by the principal investigators and from informed sources.

The objectives of the study

The objectives of the basic study and complementary surveys were to describe:

- Patterns of breast-feeding among specific social groups in selected areas of the world
- Relationships between patterns of breast-feeding, supplementary feeding, and various maternal, family, and socioeconomic characteristics
- The relationship between breast-feeding and reproduction, including the return of menstruation
- The views of mothers on breast-feeding and its duration, their reasons for not breast-feeding or discontinuing breast-feeding, and their knowledge of commercial and other baby foods
- Ways in which health services were organized with reference to maternal and infant care and infant feeding, as well as the nature and extent of legislation as it might affect maternity leave and breast-feeding
- The ways and extent to which industrially processed infant foods were marketed in the areas studied.

Location of basic study and complementary surveys

The countries included in the study were selected so as to provide a broad spectrum of geographical, ecological, and cultural characteristics; emphasis was placed on obtaining information on breast-feeding and social conditions in developing countries. Chile, Ethiopia, Guatemala, India, Nigeria, the Philippines, and Zaire provided examples of varying conditions in developing countries, and Hungary and Sweden of conditions in more industrialized societies.

Lebanon was initially also included, but local events prevented the completion of the study there.

The organization and implementation of the field work were carried out between 1975 and the spring of 1978. In Ethiopia, Guatemala, and Nigeria, owing to unforseeable problems, there were delays and interruptions in the field work, lasting in some cases for 4–12 months.

Collaborating centres in each of the nine countries were chosen for their experience with similar types of research, their interest in and capacity to undertake the work, and their access to population groups of the types outlined below.

Population groups studied

Because breast-feeding and infant-feeding behaviour in general are known to be influenced by socioeconomic, family, and especially maternal background, it was decided to seek, within each country, groups exemplifying a wide variety of conditions and characteristics. At the same time, because national populations are rarely sufficiently homogeneous for "national" samples to have more than symbolic value, while the technical difficulties of obtaining nationally representative samples are formidable, the principal investigators in the selected countries were asked to choose, on the basis of their knowledge of the national situation, groups that would serve as reasonably typical examples of the circumstances prevailing in their areas.

In each country the aim was to study three main population groups selected by the principal investigator, according to the following characteristics:

Group A: Economically advantaged, educated families in an urban area
Group C: Poor and usually poorly educated families in an urban area
Group R: Families in rural areas, usually following a traditional way of life and often dependent on subsistence agriculture and local marketing.

It was not considered feasible to propose strict conditions that could be imposed on all the groups to be studied or that would be equally applicable in all countries. Thus the principal investigators were asked to use their discretion in adapting the general definitions outlined above to local circumstances.

In both India and Nigeria, the principal investigators felt it appropriate also to include in the study an urban middle-income group (*Group B*). In Sweden, on the other hand, it was not possible to identify an urban-poor group and the characteristics of the urban and rural populations were so similar that they were ultimately combined in the analyses. In Hungary, where socioeconomic differences were also difficult to define, groups were chosen to represent Budapest, towns, and villages respectively; these, too, were also ultimately combined in the analyses. The rural (R) group in Guatemala was composed, in equal proportions, of Ladinos and

Amerindians; sample numbers did not permit these two groups to be analysed separately, but some differences between them are mentioned in the text.

Research questionnaires

A task force, composed of the principal investigators, WHO staff, and advisors, developed two main questionnaires, A and B,[1] for use in all the countries. There were pretested in draft form in English, French, and Spanish in the countries participating in the study.

Questionnaire A was designed to provide background information on the communities from which the groups to be studied were drawn. It was completed by the principal investigators and informed sources.

Questionnaire B was designed for use in interviews with mothers to record information on the social characteristics of families, circumstances of pregnancy and delivery, feeding histories and the reasons behind them, and attitudes to breast-feeding, as well as data on reproduction and family planning practices.

Part I of Questionnaire B, dealing with the background of the mothers and families and with feeding and family planning practices, was mandatory; most items were precoded. Part II, which concerns maternal opinions about breast-feeding, was designed as an optional part of the interview, but, in practice, was invariably completed too; questions in this part were more open-ended.

In addition to Questionnaires A and B, *data collection guides*[2] were developed for the collection of information on (*a*) the organization of maternity and paediatric services, (*b*) the extent to which training courses for health personnel covered the problems of breast-feeding, and (*c*) social and health legislation relevant to maternity and early infant care. A survey of marketing practices involving interviews with the headquarters and field-level staff of infant food companies, as well as field observations, was also undertaken and is further explained in Chapter 10.

Training of interviewers

All interviewers were locally recruited so as to be familiar with the local setting and its sociocultural characteristics. They were trained by the principal investigators and taught the use of a portable scale for weighing the index children. Throughout the data collection phase, regular sessions were held at which interviewers could report to the principal investigator any problems experienced in locating respondents and the use of the questionnaire.

---

[1] See Annex 2.

[2] See Annex 3.

Mothers were interviewed in their homes in their own language or dialect. At the time of the interview, the index child was weighed by the interviewer. The interview procedures that were followed and the way in which questionnaires were completed were systematically checked for reliability during the data collection period.

Information from mothers on birth weight was, whenever possible, checked with hospital or other available records.

Sampling methods and sample sizes

Since longitudinal studies are costly in both time and resources and, for practical reasons, must be undertaken with relatively small samples, cross-sectional studies were carried out in all nine countries.

Table 1. Distribution of mother–child pairs by country and population group

Country	Group[a]	No. of pairs	Total
Ethiopia	A	292	
	C	591	
	R	594	1 477
Nigeria	A	235	
	B	577	
	C	636	
	R	668	2 116
Zaire	A	595	
	C	598	
	R	589	1 782
Chile	A	295	
	C	296	
	R	443	1 034
Guatemala	A	591	
	C	594	
	R	600	1 785
India	A	863	
	B	994	
	C	980	
	R	1 185	4 022
Philippines	A	495	
	C	793	
	R	808	2 096
Hungary	all	7 950	7 950
Sweden	all	595	595
Total	25 groups		22 857

[a] A = economically advantaged. B = urban middle income. C = urban poor. R = rural.

The studies were designed to cover up to two years of infant feeding. However, in some groups in which breast-feeding was known to be rarely so prolonged, the period of study was curtailed. Thus, for example, in Hungary and Sweden the study was designed to cover 12 months.

Because the prevalence and duration of breast-feeding were anticipated to vary considerably, quota sampling was felt to be the most appropriate and feasible method; as a practicable minimum, 25 mother-and-child pairs were selected within each completed month of child age.

In all nearly 23 000 mother-and-child pairs were studied. The distribution of the pairs by country and population group is shown in Table 1.

Three alternative sampling frames were recommended in order to allow for local circumstances and possibilities. The first involved the utilization of birth records; the second, area sampling using a street index; and the third (the least recommended because of its selectivity) the use of hospital records.

Analysis of data

Copies of all data were sent to WHO headquarters, Geneva, where they were checked for consistency and analysed according to a standard procedure. The principal investigators were also free to undertake their own data analyses as required for local purposes.

In principle, three main analyses were undertaken: (*a*) examination of the relationships between breast-feeding patterns and a number of co-variables within the selected groups; (*b*) comparisons between groups within countries; (*c*) comparisons between countries and groups. For convenience, however, (*a*) and (*b*) were ultimately combined.

Groups of an apparently similar nature (e.g., the urban poor in different countries) usually represented very different cultures and standards of living, and comparisons between countries are therefore only descriptive.

Because of their special characteristics, multiple births were excluded from the analyses.

Constraints on interpretation

1. The groups that were studied are drawn from various countries and represent a wide range of socioeconomic and cultural circumstances. While they serve to illustrate aspects of breast-feeding behaviour, generalizations as to national patterns are possible only where no differences between groups exist, as in Hungary and Sweden.

2. Many of the tables and graphs in the report give the prevalence of breast-feeding by time, but it must be borne in mind that the information was collected on a cross-sectional basis and that trends in time do not represent the progress of any particular cohort of mothers and their babies.

3. The information obtained during interviews at different child ages falls into two categories. In the first category, the information gathered is not dependent on the timing of the interview: for example, the mother's educational attainment and the child's weight at birth. In the second category, the information is time-dependent; for example, the figures for prevalence of breast-feeding, as determined from responses to the question "Are you breast-feeding now?", depend upon exactly when the question was asked. The second type of information will generally be more reliable.

The reliability of information on past events also depends upon the nature of the question asked and the duration of recall. In some communities, past events are often recalled by reference to other past events—for example, a festival—and the concept of calendar time may be unfamiliar. This may affect the precision of time-specific information.

With respect to this, two recall questions are of special importance: (*a*) How old was the child when breast-feeding was stopped? (*b*) How old was the child when the mother's menstrual period returned? Little can be done to check the reliability of answers to such questions, but comparisons can be made of responses obtained by recall with "here-and-now" prevalence data relating to the situation at the time of interview.

In fact, the prevalence data that were derived from recall information were found to be in reasonable agreement with strictly cross-sectional observations. It can, therefore, be assumed that the analyses based on recalled data (which involved larger numbers of responses) are likely to lead to appropriate conclusions.

4. It is necessary to guard against two types of spurious association that can arise when interpreting data of the kind gathered in the study.

The first is connected with the fact that samples are not homogeneous in terms of the characteristics being considered. For example, the fact that economically advantaged women have small families and also breast-feed for shorter periods than poor women, who have large families and breast-feed for much longer, would make it appear that there is a causal relationship between family size and breast-feeding, when in fact both are determined by the different life-styles of the two groups. In the present study, groups were deliberately polarized for socioeconomic characteristics and, by inference, for associated breast-feeding and family-size characteristics. If such groups were to be amalgated (which they should not be), spurious associations of the type described above would be almost inevitable.

A second type of spurious association can arise when pairs of events that change with time in the same or an opposite direction are considered; for example, when the prevalence of breast-feeding among mothers who go out to work is compared with that among mothers who remain at home. If, in order to increase the numbers available, infants are grouped into wide age-ranges, it is almost inevitable that this will point to the fact that mothers going out to work breast-feed less often. This will happen even if there is no real association; the prevalence of breast-feeding falls with increasing child age, and the prevalence of mothers going out to work increases.

Although for ease of presentation fairly wide age-ranges have been established in the tabulations that follow, care has been taken not to create such spurious associations. When an association is presented that may be due to a spurious correlation, a caveat is appended.

Presentation of results

All *percentages* cited in the text or the tables that follow were calculated on the data before rounding. Thus they may not always add up to the total given.

The *age groups* used refer to the age of the child in completed months. Thus, for example the group aged 2 months will include all those aged at least 2 months but not yet 3 months and will on average be aged 2.5 months. The exceptions to this rule are Hungary and Chile, for which the exact ages are indicated.

Blank spaces in *tables* mean that no information was available or that there were too few observations (usually fewer than 10) to make the figures meaningful. By contrast a zero means "none", unless otherwise stated. Figures in parentheses indicate the number of mothers or children. Unless otherwise stated, all data in the tables are from the study findings.

Explanations of terms

Breast-milk substitute means an infant formula or any other food used as a replacement for breast-milk.

Infant formula means a marketed food preparation specially formulated to satisfy the nutritional requirements of an infant up to between 4 and 6 months of age and adapted to its physiological characteristics.

Index child means a mother's youngest child.

Significant difference: this term is used throughout the report in its statistical sense.

3. Characteristics of the communities studied

This chapter summarizes the background information on the communities to which the mothers under study belonged. The information was provided by local informed sources and reported by the principal investigators in Questionnaire A (see Annex 2).

Ethiopia

The main urban groups studied are from Addis Ababa, Akaki (an industrial area adjacent to Addis Ababa) and Zebu Zeit; the rural group belongs to the province of Kembata in the Shoa Region.

The urban population is ethnically heterogeneous and includes most of the major national groups; although there is also a relatively large Moslem population, Christianity is the main religion. The ethnic composition of the rural group studied is primarily Kembata and Hadiya, and Christianity is the main religion in the area concerned.

Socioeconomic background. In the economically advantaged group, most wage-earners are in the civil service or private business; their monthly incomes ranged between US $300 and US $1750. Among the urban-poor group, factory work, unskilled work, and petty trading are the principal occupations, and monthly incomes ranged between US $15 and US $150. Subsistence farming and petty trading constitute the main occupations in the rural area, where it was difficult to assess income. The level of illiteracy is high among both the urban-poor and rural populations.

In general, the standard of housing in the economically advantaged areas is good and most homes have all modern amenities. The urban-poor and rural areas are characterized by poor-quality housing; overcrowding is common and sanitation inadequate; few homes have piped water or toilet facilities, and waste disposal systems are invariably unable to meet community needs.

Nutrition. Dietary patterns vary considerably between the groups studied. Among the economically advantaged, a wide variety of foods, including meat and dairy products, is regularly consumed. In the other two groups, the diet is considerably more restricted: cereals such as teff, wheat, maize, and barley, together with legumes and tubers, are the staple foods, and meat and dairy products are consumed only infrequently.

During the period of the study, food was in short supply.

Breast-milk substitutes. Shops, kiosks, and pharmacies in the urban area retail a variety of breast-milk substitutes (17 brands of infant formula are available). While the promotion of commercial infant foods is not intensive, they are advertised through the mass media and street sale campaigns are not infrequent.

Health services. Health services for the urban population are available through hospitals and maternal and child health clinics, but traditional healers are also patronized by all social groups. In the rural area, the hospital closest to the group studied is 45 km away and the only other health care service is a local smallpox eradication programme.

Nigeria

The urban groups studied are from Ibadan; the rural group is made up of samples from two villages with a total population of approximately 2500. With the exception of the urban-poor group, which includes a large number of Igbira migrants, the background of the groups was primarily Yoruba.

Christianity is the main religion among the economically advantaged and middle-income groups, but in the urban-poor group indigenous religions predominate. About 70% of the rural study population is Muslim, 10% is Christian, and the remainder follow traditional African religions.

Among recent migrants to the city and in the rural areas, polygamy continues to be common.

Socioeconomic background. Most of the economically advantaged urban population work in the civil service or the teaching profession, with monthly incomes ranging between US $600 and US $1150. The main occupations of the middle-income groups are teaching, clerical work, and nursing; their incomes range between US $140 and US $250 per month. Overall, the level of education in the urban areas is high and illiteracy is rare. In the old part of the city, petty trading and skilled manual work are the main sources of employment and the *per capita* income among the urban poor is less than US $80 a month. The literacy rate is high among the Christian population but low among the remainder of the urban-poor population; the situation is the same in the periurban, newly settled areas, where incomes rarely exceed US $65 per month.

The economic basis of the rural area is subsistence farming (maize, yam, and cassava) and commercial farming (cocoa, maize). It was difficult to estimate a monthly income in this area since the money flow varies seasonally.

The standard of housing in economically advantaged areas is good, with adequate water supply and sound waste disposal and sanitation. In middle-income areas, sanitation and waste disposal are much less adequate and water has to be drawn from standpipes.

Houses in the older, more traditional area of the city are small and usually overcrowded; there is no electricity, ventilation is generally poor, and sanitation facilities are limited; water is taken from standpipes. In the periurban area too, overcrowding is common, most houses being occupied by several families who share cooking facilities. Sanitation is poor; water is drawn from standpipes and in some cases from streams. In the rural communities, environmental sanitation is again poor and water tends to be drawn mainly from streams; there is no system of organized waste disposal.

Nutrition. Among economically advantaged families, the diet usually includes meat, fish, eggs, dairy produce, vegetables, fruit, and a variety of cereals. In low-income groups, maize, beans and green vegetables are the staple foods; meat may be available no more than once a week, and fish two to three times a week. Dairy products, root vegetables, and eggs are less common.

In the rural areas, the daily family diet usually includes maize, green vegetables, and roots such as cassava and yams; pulses (beans and locust beans) are less frequently consumed and beef and fish are probably eaten only once a week.

Breast-milk substitutes. A wide variety of breast-milk substitutes is marketed in Nigeria through pharmacies, food stores, kiosks, supermarkets, and grocery shops. Promotion is intensive. In Ibadan breast-milk substitutes are advertised through newspapers, radio, television, and promotional visits by salesmen to health centres, prenatal clinics, and well-baby clinics. In the rural area there is intensive sales promotion of such products on village market-days. In both the urban and rural areas, free samples are regularly given away as part of publicity campaigns.

Health services. A university teaching hospital, two general hospitals, 12 general practices, and a number of maternal and child health centres are located in or close to the areas from which the urban economically advantaged group was drawn.

The urban-poor groups are all located within about 3 km of a maternal and child health centre; the rural group is served by two health centres.

Zaire

The three groups studied were drawn from the Kivu region. The population of Bukavu, the urban area, is ethnically heterogeneous: 54% Shi, 19% Rega, and 5% Havu, the remainding 22% consisting of a variety of peoples from other parts of Zaire. The rural area, where 90% of the inhabitants are Shi, has the most homogeneous population.

Socioeconomic background. It is estimated that about 60% of the urban population have a monthly income of less than US $60 and that about 30%

earn less than US $20 per month. School enrolment is high and, even in the low-income areas of the city, about 50% of children in the 6–14 year old age group attend school.

In the rural area, where women constitute the mainstay of the agricultural labour force, about 80% of the adult population is involved in subsistence farming; another 10% work on plantations, and the remainder are artisans. The *per capita* income may be as low as US $60 per annum, of which only one quarter is in the form of monetary revenue. Less than 25% of the adult population have attended school, and illiteracy is common.

Within the residential district and the planned city of Bukavu district, houses, although small, are generally of good quality; most homes have piped water and environmental sanitation is generally good. In the poorer areas of the city, the standard of housing is low, while the water supply and waste disposal systems are on the whole inadequate and unable to meet the needs of the community.

In the rural area, houses tend to be dispersed and there are few well-defined villages. It is usual for heads of households to live alone and for mothers and young children to inhabit a second house. In some cases there may also be a third house for a grandfather and guests, and a fourth for adolescent children, as well as a hut reserved for grandmothers and prepubertal children. Water supply and sanitation in the rural area are poor.

Nutrition. Although the range of foods grown in the area is broad, the ones most frequently consumed are beans, sweet potato, manioc, and bananas (banana beer is a popular drink). Consumption of animal products is low and, while the population is essentially a pastoral one, little milk is consumed by either adults or children.

There is no period of the year during which energy intake is particularly low, but there is considerable fluctuation in protein intake and, especially during October-December, there is a significant protein shortage.

Breast-milk substitutes. Breast-milk substitutes are available in food stores in the urban area; in the rural area, powdered milk is available, although it is not expressly sold as baby food. There is little evidence of intensive advertising of breast-milk substitutes.

Health services. The health services available vary considerably in type from one area to another. In the urban area, for example, they are part of the national health system, but in the rural area studied, services are provided by a number of international and nongovernment agencies.

Chile

The economically advantaged group studied is from residential areas in the eastern part of Santiago, and the urban-poor group from two areas to the north of Santiago. The rural group is located about 70 km from Santiago.

The urban economically advantaged group is primarily of European origin, and the urban-poor and rural groups are of mixed Spanish and Indian (Mapuche) origin.

Socioeconomic background. Most heads of households in the economically advantaged group are employed in high-level technical and executive positions. Information on income levels is not available. In the urban-poor group, in which the main sources of employment are construction and factory work, the minimum income is estimated to be approximately US $32 per month. About 90 % of the total adult urban population is estimated to be literate.

In the rural areas market-gardening and mining (often augmented by subsistence farming) are the main sources of employment. The higher income levels are not known, but the lower levels are estimated at US $30 a month. The illiteracy rate in the rural areas is estimated to be about 65 %.

Housing in the economically advantaged areas is of a high standard, and sanitation and water supply services are well maintained. In the urban-poor areas, much of the housing is government-sponsored and public services are generally good; piped water is available to most homes but, where it is not available, water is drawn from neighbourhood wells or street standpipes. Houses in the rural area are usually small and built of adobe, and overcrowding is not uncommon. Although there is a good network of piped water, there are still areas where it is necessary to draw water from wells and standpipes. Waste disposal facilities are generally poor.

Nutrition. In the economically advantaged group, cereals such as rice, together with a wide range of vegetables, fruit, meat, and dairy products, are part of the regular diet. Among the urban poor, rice and vegetables are common, but such foods as fruit, root vegetables, and fish are less frequently available and meat and beans are consumed only once a month. In the rural areas the situation is similar; meat is consumed very infrequently and fish even more rarely. The availability of food, moreover, tends to be more seasonally determined than in the urban communities.

Breast-milk substitutes. Breast-milk substitutes are widely available in the urban areas through pharmacies. There is some advertising through pharmacies, but in general it is not intensive.

Health services. In the case of the economically advantaged group, most health care is of a private nature and financed through work or private insurance schemes. The urban poor tend primarily to use maternal and child health centres closely linked to the hospital system of the national health service. In the rural area studied there is a small hospital with six paediatric beds, four internal medicine beds, and provision for ambulatory care.

Guatemala

The urban groups—both the economically advantaged and the poor—were selected from within Guatemala City, and the rural group from small highland communities located 35–55 km away. The population of Guatemala is composed of two main ethnic groups – Ladinos who are predominantly of European descent and are Spanish-speaking, and Indians who are indigenous to Guatemala and maintain their own languages and distinct life-style. The urban groups studied were predominantly Ladino, whereas the rural sample contained both Ladino and Indian groups. There is little residential integration between the two ethnic groups in the rural areas, and Ladinos and Indians were drawn from different villages.

Socioeconomic background. In the economically advantaged group, in which the principal sources of employment are professional activity, private business, and skilled trades, the average family income is about US $600 per month. The educational level is generally high, and illiteracy is virtually unknown in the adult population.

The main occupations in the urban-poor areas are skilled manual work, unskilled labour, and "low-level" employment in government offices; here the average monthly income is of the order of US $20 per person. Illiteracy is again uncommon.

In the rural communities, subsistence farming is common but land holdings are small and productivity is low. Although monthly incomes may be in the range of US $10 per person, seasonal fluctuations often bring them considerably lower. Illiteracy is common.

Standards of housing in the urban economically advantaged areas are good; most homes are of modern construction and have modern amenities and good sanitation. The low-income dwellings usually consist of large, cheaply constructed houses, in which families rent rooms, or shanty houses on the periphery of the city. Neighbourhoods are crowded; about a third of the population draws its water from neighbourhood taps; roads are often unpaved and, in the wet season, difficult to use; latrines and toilets are usually located between the houses but there is no organized system for the disposal of solid wastes.

Houses in the rural areas are usually of adobe, with mud floors. In the Ladino villages, they are more dispersed than in the Indian communities and tend to have more amenities, nevertheless, in many areas water has to be drawn from wells or neighbourhood taps. The quality of water throughout the rural area is poor and families are encouraged to boil all water intended for drinking or cooking. There is no organized system of waste disposal.

Nutrition. Corn tortillas, wheat bread, rice, noodles, and black beans are staple foods throughout Guatemala, but among the economically advantaged these are regularly complemented by dairy produce, meat, chicken, and green vegetables.

In the rural areas tortillas and black beans are staples; rice is eaten once or twice a week. Although dairy produce, meat, chicken, and green vegetables are available, these are not effectively utilized in some areas.

Breast-milk substitutes. In the urban communities breast-milk substitutes and powdered milk are widely available through supermarkets, pharmacies, grocery shops, etc., and the range of brand products available is wide. In the rural areas, they are much less easy to come by. In the urban areas, they are intensively advertised in newspapers, on television and radio, and by posters. In addition, paediatricians are regularly visited by baby-food representatives and given free samples. In rural communities, advertising of baby foods is limited and mainly over the radio.

Health services. There are three well-equipped private hospitals, as well as several private clinics, which are used by the economically advantaged urban groups; the urban-poor area contains a large public health centre, a number of private clinics, and a large public hospital.

There are no health centres in any of the rural Ladino communities that were studied, although they are about 4 km from a hospital; all three Indian communities included in the study have health centres.

India

The study was conducted in the State of Andra Pradesh, where the urban study groups were selected from the twin cities of Hyderabad and Secunderabad. The rural group studied was drawn from the Ramannapet Block in the Nalganda District about 450 km from Hyderabad. The population is mainly composed of Hindus and Muslims; the urban area contains large numbers of immigrants from other states of India.

Socioeconomic background. Most wage-earners in the economically advantaged and middle-income groups are of the white-collar type: senior administrators and professional men, clerical and technically skilled workers. The overall level of education in both groups is high, as is the proportion of university graduates. Monthly incomes range from US $400 to US $500 among the economically advantaged; in the middle-income group, the range is US $70 to US $125.

The main occupations among the urban poor are usually of an unskilled type, e.g., driving and domestic service, although some families own small businesses, such as bicycle repair shops and roadside food stalls. Illiteracy is common among men and women. Incomes range from US $10 to US $40.

Most of the rural families are dependent on agricultural work, usually of a subsistence kind (rice, sorghum, and millet) with some commercial tobacco-growing, with daily incomes ranging from US $0.40 to US $0.70 during the high season. Illiteracy is common.

In the economically advantaged and middle-income areas, housing is modern and electricity, piped water supply, and sewage disposal systems are standard features.

In the urban-poor areas where homes are usually built of mud with roofs of asbestos or galvanized iron, interior ventilation is poor and homes are overcrowded; latrines are communal and drainage facilities generally inadequate or nonexistent. Housing conditions in the rural area are much the same; houses are of mud and brick with thatched roofs, ventilation is poor, and potable water is available only from communal wells or taps. Waste disposal facilities are generally inadequate, and stagnant water pools are common in most of the rural communities.

Nutrition. Among the upper- and middle-income groups, wheat and a variety of peas and lentils, vegetables and fruits, and milk and dairy products are part of the daily diet. Rice and wheat are the staple food of the rural poor and, although meat is not a regular part of their daily diet, they appear to prefer it to fish. Green and root vegetables are not consumed on a regular basis.

In the rural area, rice, jowar, bajra, and chick (red and green) peas are all part of the staple diet. Green and root vegetables are eaten irregularly, and the availability of fruit (banana, sitaphal) is limited. Meat, fish, and eggs are not common in the local diet, though some families eat them.

Breast-milk substitutes. A broad variety of breast-milk substitutes is widely available in the urban areas through food stores and those specializing in pharmaceutical and medical products; in the rural areas, they are available through shops located close to primary health care centres and medical supply stores.

In the city, the advertising of infant formula is carried out through the mass media and is quite intensive; in the rural areas, it is less so but regular advertisements for such products nevertheless appear in newspapers and are also carried by the radio.

Food donations from international organizations, including milk powder, are distributed through social welfare departments, hospitals, and outpatient departments to urban-poor and rural families.

Health services. The urban area of Hyderabad is served by public hospitals, but among the economically advantaged and middle-income groups there is a tendency to use private nursing homes and specialist consultancy services as well as the public hospitals. In the rural area studied, there is a 30-bed hospital and a primary health centre.

Philippines

The study covered three population groups: an economically advantaged group from Paranaque, adjacent to Manila; an urban-poor group from Pasay, within the metropolitan area of Manila; and a rural group from San Rafael on the island of Luzon.

Both the urban study groups are essentially of Indonesian-Malayan origin, although a number of the regional ethnic groups are also represented. In the rural area the population is predominantly Tagalog.

Socioeconomic background. Within the economically advantaged group, the main occupations are professional and incomes are of the order of US $300–US $700 per month. The principal occupations among the urban poor are unskilled labour and domestic service, for which incomes vary considerably, labourers earning around US $25 per month and domestic servants between US $10 and $20 per month. On the whole, school enrolment is high and illiteracy relatively uncommon in all groups. In the rural area, subsistence farming is the principal occupation and is sometimes complemented by the growing of cash crops.

The quality of housing in the economically advantaged area is good; modern amenities are common and environmental sanitation of a high standard. Conditions in the urban-poor area are characterized by poor water supply, inadequate waste disposal, environmental pollution, and overcrowding. Housing and living conditions in the rural area are somewhat better, in that there is less overcrowding and better environmental sanitation, including water supply.

Nutrition. A wide variety of foods is available throughout the country; among the economically advantaged group, the diet is varied and regularly includes meat, fish, and vegetables. For the urban poor, rice is a staple food; meat is rarely consumed, but fish is a relatively common part of the diet. A more varied diet, with a broader selection of vegetables and more frequent consumption of fish, is found in the rural communities.

Breast-milk substitutes. Breast-milk substitutes are widely available to all three groups studied. In the urban communties particularly, they are carried by groceries, pharmacies, and supermarkets. Advertising is intensive, promotion being carried out through all the available media and by visits of baby-food representatives to homes and health services. Free samples are provided through the health services.

Health services. In the urban economically advantaged community, there are two general hospitals and a number of health centres, but most of the health care services used by this group are private. In the urban-poor community, health centres are the source of most care but there is also a domiciliary obstetrical service. Rural health units provide most of the care available to the population of San Rafael.

Hungary

Because of the difficulty of characterizing the population in terms of socioeconomic differences, study groups were selected on the basis of residential/ecological background: "large urban centre" (Budapest), "towns", and "rural communities".

All groups studied are predominantly of Hungarian descent. Approximately two-thirds of the population are Catholic, the remainder Protestant.

Socioeconomic background. Side by side with industry, agriculture (both subsistence and commercial) still occupies an important place in the economy. There is considerable internal migration of labour, both temporary and permanent, all the year round. The average monthly income ranges from US $140 for village workers to US $200 for professionals. Education is universal and illiteracy uncommon.

Housing characteristics do not vary much between rural and urban areas. Practically all homes have electricity, and about half of them are connected to piped water supplies. Environmental sanitation is, in general, good.

Nutrition. A wide range of foods is available throughout the year; cereals, dairy products, and pork are the staple foods.

Breast-milk substitutes. Breast-milk substitutes are available in most pharmacies and food shops, and some products are also occasionally provided free through maternal and child health centres; in some cases a medical prescription is required. Diluted cow's milk is also used for infant feeding.

Health services. Health care services are provided by the state and are free of charge. All social groups have easy access to hospitals, policlinics, and health centres.

Sweden

The study was carried out in the county of Uppsala. Two groups were included, one an urban sample drawn from the city of Uppsala, the other a rural sample from a combination of several small villages and communities with populations ranging between 1000 and 3000 inhabitants and from the town of Tierp.

The majority of the population is of Swedish origin and, for the most part, Lutheran. About 8 % of the population is composed of immigrants, mainly from southern Europe.

Socioeconomic background. The city of Uppsala is an administrative, educational, and trade centre, and the occupational backgrounds of the inhabitants are varied. In the rural area, which is primarily agricultural, practically all farming is commercial; the main crops are wheat, rye, barley, oats, and oil-seed.

At the time of the study, the minimum income for wage-earners was of the order of US $700 per month; at the upper level of the scale, it could reach about US $3500 per month. Taxation on earnings is relatively high, but all education and medical care services are free and there is a broad range of social services.

It is estimated that all children of school age are enrolled in schools, and illiteracy is almost unknown.

There is little variation in the quality of housing or the amenities available to urban and rural populations. The main differences are found in the higher frequency of private residences or individual houses in the rural areas, as opposed to apartment dwellings in the city. The level of environmental sanitation and the quality of water supplies is, in general, high.

Nutrition. A broad variety of foods is available all year round. As well as the basic cereals (wheat, rye, oats, barley), legumes, vegetables, and dairy products are produced locally, and there is a broad selection of fruit and greens from other parts of Europe. Meat (pork, lamb, beef, and chicken) is commonly eaten, as are different varieties of fish.

Breast-milk substitutes. Breast-milk substitutes and commercially prepared baby foods are sold in most grocery stores, supermarkets, and pharmacies. Advertising of baby foods, in particular breast-milk substitutes, however, is limited according to a national code of ethics. Advertisements for breast-milk substitutes, for example, are limited to professional periodicals and journals, but displays of dummy boxes of infant-food products are permitted at health centres, and breast-milk substitutes are frequently mentioned in the booklets on child care and nutrition products distributed by infant-food manufacturers.

Health services. A 2000-bed university hospital is located in Uppsala, and transport services from the rural communities to Uppsala are good. All the communities included in the study have convenient access to child health centres. Maternity and child health services cover all infants and children up to the age of seven.

4. Prevalence and duration of breast-feeding

In each of the population groups studied, mothers were asked if they were breast-feeding their respective index (i.e., youngest) children at the time of the interview. Those who replied in the negative were asked if the infants in question had ever been breast-fed, and if so, for how many months. This chapter presents a summary of the cross-sectional (point-prevalence) and recalled information given in response to this and other questions concerning the pattern of breast-feeding, including reasons for not breast-feeding or for stopping breast-feeding, together with mothers' views on how long breast-feeding should be continued and on the need for privacy when breast-feeding.

Overall prevalence of breast-feeding

The proportions of mothers in each country and population group who reported ever breast-feeding the index children are shown in Table 2 and Fig. 1. In Nigeria and Zaire, breast-feeding was universal among all groups as it was among the rural groups in India and Ethiopia. Otherwise, its prevalence appeared to be related to socioeconomic background. Except in Hungary and Sweden, breast-feeding was notably more common in rural than urban areas, and within the urban populations it was more prevalent among the poor than among the economically advantaged.

It is particularly noteworthy that a large proportion of mothers in the economically advantaged groups in the Philippines and Guatemala reported that they had never breast-fed the index children; the proportions for these groups were respectively 10 and 7 times higher than those for Hungarian mothers, and also 5 and 4 times higher than those for Swedish mothers. Even among urban-poor mothers in the Philippines, Guatemala, and Chile, the proportions not breast-feeding were higher than in either Hungary or Sweden.

In general breast-feeding was more common in the C (urban-poor) groups than in the A (economically advantaged) groups, and more common in the R (rural) groups than in the C groups.

Mothers' reasons for not breast-feeding were given in answer to an open-ended question. Some mothers gave more than one reason without indicating priorities, but since the principal consideration was the type and

Table 2. Percentage of mothers who had ever breast-fed index children

Country	Group[a]	Percentage
Ethiopia	A	91
	C	97
	R	100
Nigeria	A	100
	B	100
	C	100
	R	100
Zaire	A	100
	C	100
	R	100
Chile	A	93
	C	92
	R	95
Guatemala	A	77
	C	91
	R	98
India	A	96
	B	96
	C	99
	R	100
Philippines	A	68
	C	85
	R	94
Hungary	all	97
Sweden	all	93

[a] See footnote to Table 1.

range of reasons mothers gave, all their responses were considered. The most common overall reason was "lack of" or "insufficient" milk. Among the urban economically advantaged and middle-income groups in India, and among the urban poor of Chile and the Philippines, for example, this was mentioned in over half of the responses. In the rural group in Chile, "child sick" was the most frequent reason; in India among the B group (urban middle-income) a frequent reason was that the mother had been ill (see also Annex 1, Table A1).

Fig. 1. Percentage of women who had ever breast-fed index children, by country and socioeconomic group

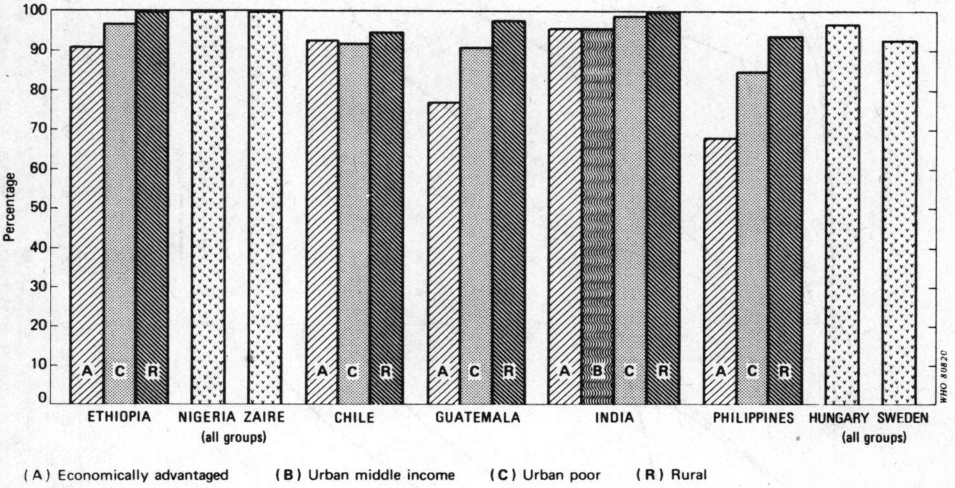

Proportion of mothers breast-feeding, by age of child

Fig. 2 gives the prevalence of breast-feeding by age of child for the different groups studied; the curves have been smoothed using the larger numbers provided by retrospective information from mothers who were no longer breast-feeding at the time they were interviewed.

It is interesting that in the two population groups in which there were the highest proportions of mothers who never breast-fed the general duration of breast-feeding among those that did also tended to be shorter; in the Philippines and Guatemala, for example, over 50 % of mothers in the A group had weaned their infants by about the second month, a pattern that contrasts sharply with that observed in Nigeria, Zaire, and India.

Among the urban-poor groups the shortest duration of breast-feeding was in Chile where, by the age of 6 months, over 50 % of infants had been weaned; next came the Philippines and Guatemala where two-thirds of all infants had been weaned by the age of 6 months.

As shown in Fig. 3, the observed patterns of breast-feeding duration fall into three quite distinct categories. It will be shown later that the same categories apply to the patterns of post-partum return of menstruation.

In Category I, in which the prevalence of breast-feeding falls steeply with child age, are all A groups (with the exception of those in India and Zaire), and all mothers in Hungary and Sweden. The first category also includes the C group from Chile, in which breast-feeding tended to be less common than among the economically advantaged. In none of the groups that fall into Category I was the prevalence of breast-feeding at 6 months higher

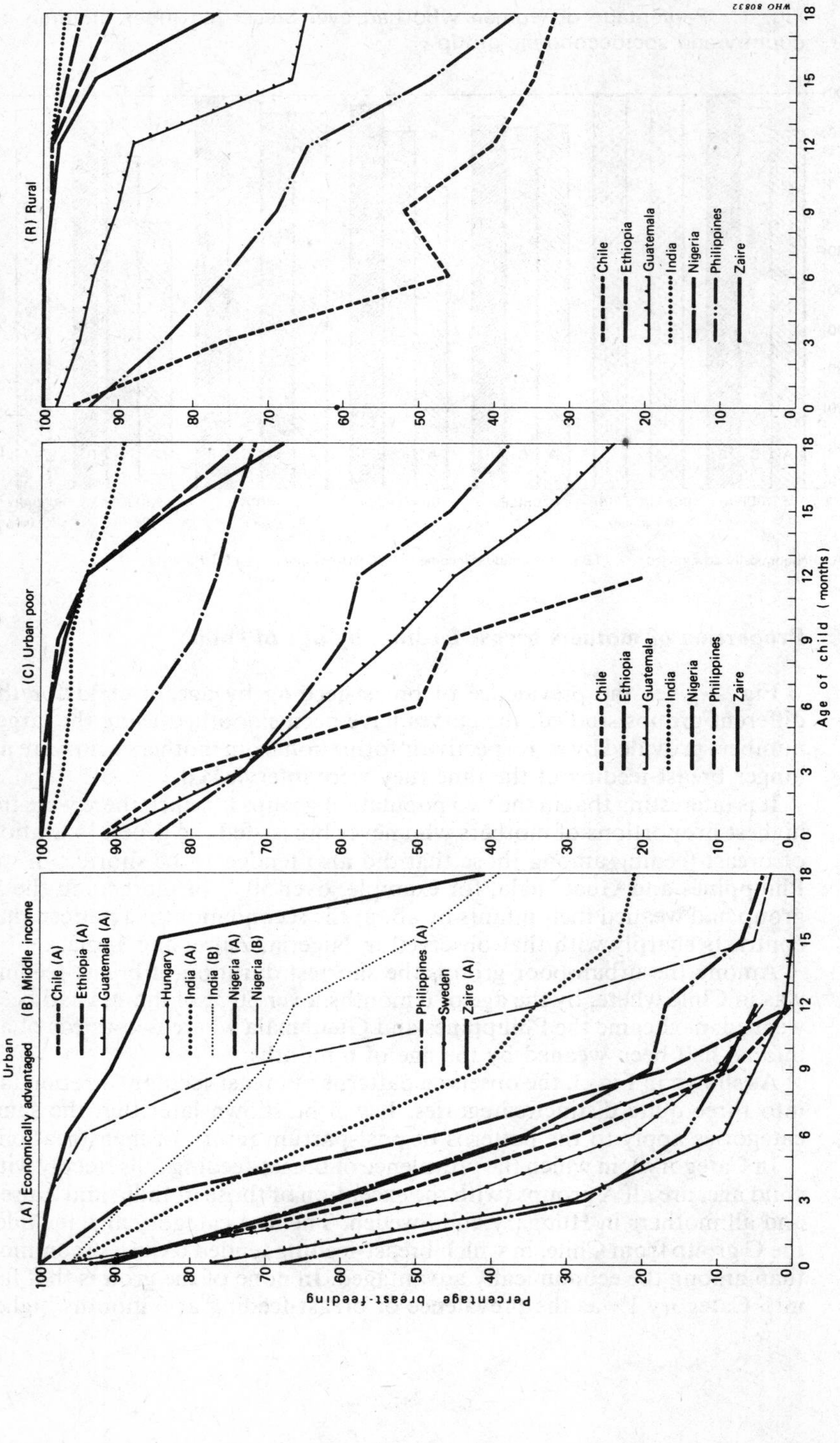

Fig. 2. Percentage of mothers breast-feeding, by age of child, country, and socioeconomic group

Fig. 3. Percentage of mothers breast-feeding, by age of child and population group (three categories)

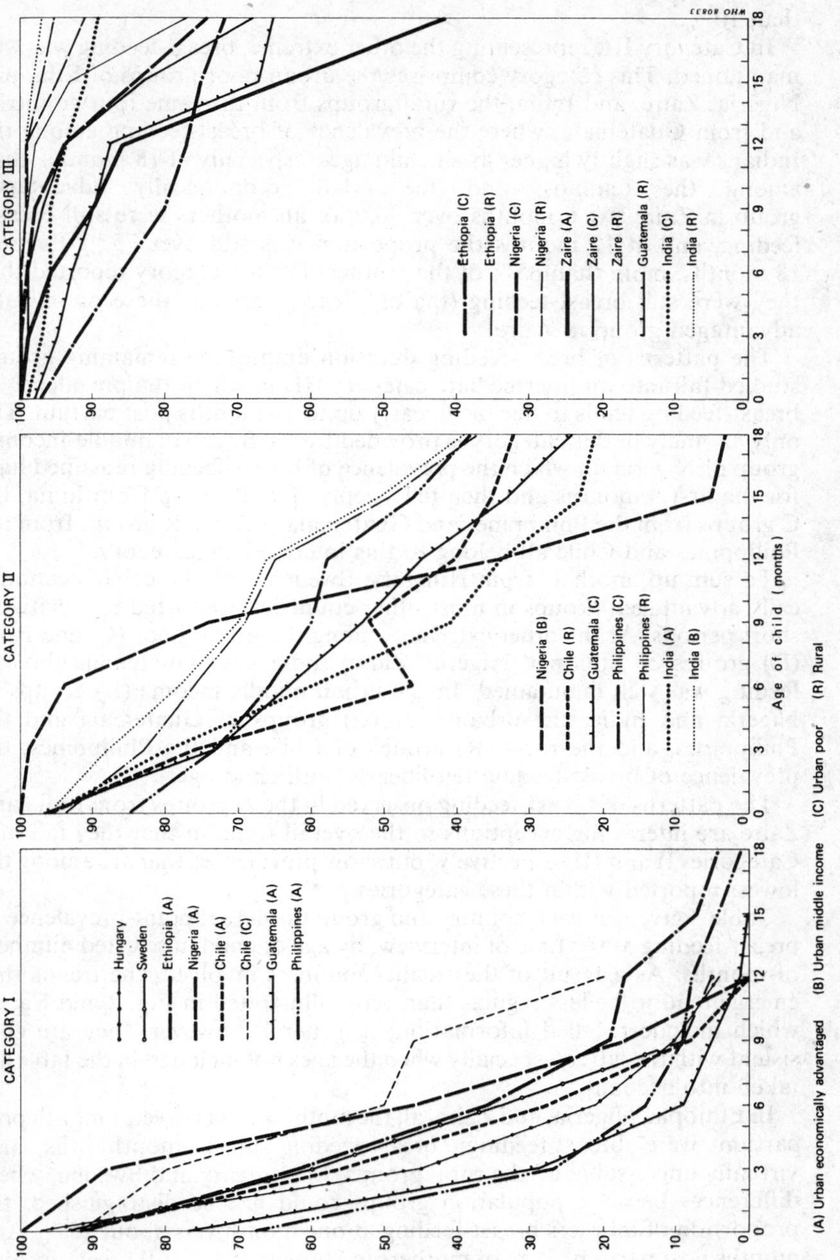

than 50 %; and at 12 months only two groups had a prevalence of more than 10 %.

In Category III, representing the other extreme, breast-feeding was well maintained. This category comprises the urban-poor groups of Ethiopia, Nigeria, Zaire, and India; the rural groups from the same four countries and from Guatemala, where the prevalence of breast-feeding among the Indians was slightly higher at all child ages, especially at 18 months, than among the Ladinos; and the urban economically advantaged group in Zaire. At 6 months over 90 % of all mothers were still breast-feeding, and at 12 months the proportion was still over 75 %. Even at 18 months, more than 65 % of the mothers in this category reported that they were still breast-feeding (the only exception was the economically advantaged group in Zaire).

The patterns of breast-feeding duration among the remaining groups studied fall into an intermediate category (II) in which the prevalence of breast-feeding tends to decline linearly up to 18 months post partum. The only anomaly in this category is provided by the B (urban middle-income) group of Nigeria, in which the prevalence of breast-feeding remained high for the first 9 months and then fell steeply. The B group from India, the C groups from the Philippines and Guatemala, and the R groups from the Philippines and Chile all belong to this intermediate category.

To sum up, mothers from Hungary, Sweden, and the urban economically advantaged groups in most other countries breast-fed for relatively short periods. At the other extreme, among the urban poor (C) and rural (R) groups of Ethiopia, Nigeria, Zaire, India, and Guatemala, breast-feeding was well maintained. In the urban middle-income (B) groups of Nigeria and India, the urban-poor (C) groups of Guatemala and the Philippines, and the rural (R) groups of Chile and the Philippines, the prevalence of breast-feeding fell linearly with child age.

The patterns of breast-feeding observed in the A groups from India and Zaire are interesting exceptions to the overall trend in that they fall into Categories II and III respectively, but show prevalences that are among the lowest reported within these categories.

Table 3 gives for each country and group the actual point-prevalence of breast-feeding at the time of interview, by age of child in selected numbers of months. As a result of the smaller numbers involved, the trends that emerge tend to be less regular than those illustrated in Fig. 2 and Fig. 3, which include recalled information; in general, however, they are consistent with the latter, especially when the ages not included in the table are taken into account.

In Ethiopia, Nigeria, and Zaire, all the mothers interviewed 1 month post partum were breast-feeding; breast-feeding at 1 month was also virtually universal in all the rural groups. In Hungary and Sweden, where differences between population groups could not be distinguished, the proportion of mothers breast-feeding at one month was about 75 %. At 6 months post partum, 21 % of mothers in Hungary were still breast-feeding and in Sweden the proportion was 34 %.

Table 3. Percentage of mothers breast-feeding at time of interview, by age of child*

Country	Group[a]	Age of child (months) 1	3	6	9	12	15	18
		%	%	%	%	%	%	%
Ethiopia	A		59 (22)	35 (17)	29 (14)		0 (13)	8 (13)
	C	100 (36)	87 (32)	81 (27)	81 (31)	76 (37)	73 (15)	70 (20)
	R	100 (23)	100 (29)	100 (17)	100 (48)	98 (46)	100 (18)	97 (29)
Nigeria	A	100 (20)	96 (23)	32 (19)	20 (20)	0 (20)		
	B	100 (25)	100 (23)	91 (23)	68 (22)	22 (23)	4 (23)	0 (22)
	C	100 (25)	100 (26)	97 (36)	100 (31)	97 (29)	96 (25)	79 (24)
	R	100 (26)	100 (27)	100 (27)	100 (29)	97 (38)	96 (25)	82 (28)
Zaire	A	100 (25)	100 (25)	100 (25)	83 (24)	80 (25)	64 (25)	25 (24)
	C	100 (25)	100 (25)	100 (25)	96 (25)	84 (25)	80 (25)	56 (25)
	R	100 (25)	100 (25)	100 (25)	100 (25)	96 (24)	87 (24)	80 (25)
Chile	A	80 (25)	56 (25)	28 (25)	8 (24)	0 (23)		
	C	92 (24)	80 (25)	39 (23)	46 (24)	20 (25)		
	R	92 (25)	76 (25)	46 (24)	52 (23)	40 (25)	23 (26)	32 (25)
Guatemala	A	44 (55)	29 (42)	4 (47)	5 (22)	0 (14)	0 (10)	
	C	88 (26)	76 (25)	73 (26)	62 (26)	29 (24)	39 (28)	29 (28)
	R	95 (22)	97 (29)	97 (29)	90 (29)	82 (33)	91 (22)	61 (31)
India	A	87 (39)	84 (38)	49 (37)	47 (36)	33 (36)	18 (33)	29 (31)
	B	95 (40)	78 (41)	72 (47)	66 (47)	58 (48)	51 (35)	44 (32)
	C	97 (38)	95 (40)	88 (58)	95 (38)	93 (56)	94 (54)	80 (41)
	R	100 (50)	100 (50)	100 (55)	100 (48)	99 (85)	97 (31)	95 (59)
Philippines	A	61 (31)	27 (26)	19 (31)	5 (22)	6 (16)	13 (15)	0 (12)
	C	69 (35)	61 (46)	53 (45)	38 (29)	52 (31)	29 (38)	34 (29)
	R	92 (49)	83 (35)	89 (28)	75 (36)	63 (30)	42 (33)	42 (33)
Hungary	all	77 (615)	45 (616)	21 (763)	10 (658)	4 (630)		
Sweden	all	73 (49)	44 (50)	34 (50)	10 (49)	6 (50)[b]		

* Figures in parentheses indicate actual numbers of mothers interviewed.

[a] See footnote to Table 1.

[b] 11 months.

The lowest prevalence at one month was reported in the A groups in Guatemala (44 %) and the Philippines (61 %). By 6 months these had fallen to 5 % and 19 % respectively. These are the same two groups in which a high proportion of women reported that they did not breast-feed at all (Table 2). There was no evidence in any group studied that the sex of the children influenced the prevalence of breast-feeding.

Reasons for stopping breast-feeding

The question on reasons for stopping breast-feeding was open-ended, and mothers were allowed to give more than one response. The reasons given varied considerably and, even when the terms used by mothers in the different countries were similar, it may not necessarily follow that the meaning behind them was the same.

No analysis was possible in the case of Ethiopia because the question was not answered in a sufficiently high proportion of cases.

Up to three-quarters of the responses in Nigeria, where the median age at weaning was about 6 months in the A group, 11 months in the B group, and well over 18 months in the C and R groups, alluded to the child simply being "old enough", or old enough for the mother "to introduce solids", or to the fact that it was the "mother's decision" that the time had come to wean the child. Insufficient milk and poor sucking accounted for 10–20 % of the responses. A new pregnancy was the reason given in 13 % of cases among groups C and R, but in less than 5 % of cases in groups A and B.

In Zaire, where the median age at weaning in all groups was well over 18 months, a new pregnancy was a particularly frequent reason, being given in 33 % of cases in the A group, 51 % in the B group, and 57 % in the R group. The second most important set of reasons involved such explanations as "child too big" and "child eats well"; these accounted 35 %, 13 %, and 26 % respectively of the responses in the three groups.

Among Chilean mothers about three-quarters of the responses in all groups gave "insufficient milk" as the reason; a further 8 % to 12 % referred to poor sucking or the child's refusal to suck. About 10 % of the responses mentioned poor health of mother or child, but especially of the former. Pregnancy accounted for 3 % of the responses in the R group and slightly less of those in the A and C groups. The median age at weaning was about 4 months in the A group and about 6 months in the R and C groups.

In Guatemala "poor milk supply" was referred to in 60 % of the responses given by the A group, in which the median age at weaning was below 2 months, and in 44 % and 28 % respectively of those given by the C and R groups, in which the median ages at weaning were 10 months and well over 18 months. Poor sucking or refusal to suck was the reason advanced in 6 %, 15 %, and 19 % respectively of responses in the three groups (A, C, and R). Pregnancy was given as the reason for stopping breast-feeding in 6 % of responses in the C group and 17 % of those in the R group. In the A group, 12 % of mothers said they stopped breast-feeding "for practical reasons".

In India, where most mothers in the R group were still breast-feeding at the time of the interview, there were only 16 responses from this group, 10 of which referred to new pregnancies. Pregnancy was the reason given in 2%, 6%, and 13% of the responses in the A, B, and C groups respectively. In the same three groups, about two-thirds of the responses referred to "insufficient milk".

In the Philippines, about half the responses referred to "insufficient milk". Return to work was the reason given in 19% of responses in the A group (median age at weaning, below 2 months), and 9% of these in the C and R groups (median age at weaning, over 1 year). In the three groups, pregnancy was given as a reason in 2%, 10%, and 10% of cases respectively. Illness of the mother or the child (especially of the former) was advanced in about 12%, 22%, and 7% of the responses in the three groups.

In Hungary, where the median age at weaning was about 3 months, the most common reason (70% of the responses) for stopping breast-feeding was insufficient milk; a further 18% referred to the child's poor sucking or refusal to suck. A new pregnancy was never given as the reason.

In Sweden, where the median age at weaning was about 5 months, insufficient milk (33%) and poor sucking (24%) were again the most common reasons. Another 14% of the responses indicated that the mothers simply did not want to continue breast-feeding; 4% reported they had difficulties with their breasts or nipples. Illness of mother or child and maternal work needs each accounted for 7% of the responses. As in Hungary, pregnancy was not mentioned as a reason for stopping breast-feeding.

It is clear that the reasons advanced should be considered in the light of information on the duration of breast-feeding in the various groups. It is of interest that "insufficient milk" was given as a reason not only by rural mothers, among whom prolonged breast-feeding was common, but also by economically advantaged urban mothers who on the whole tended to breast-feed for a much shorter time.

Frequency of breast-feeding

Mothers were asked whether their babies were breast-fed "on demand", "on schedule", or according to some "other" pattern, i.e., one in which the mother met the baby's demands as her other activities permitted. Table 4 shows the percentage frequencies of these feeding patterns among mothers who were interviewed during the first and second trimesters post partum and who were still breast-feeding at the time.

The data suggest that, except in Hungary and in some of the A groups, feeding on demand was by far the most popular practice; this was especially so among rural and urban-poor mothers. In Sweden and in the Indian urban groups, a relatively high proportion of mothers said they followed "other" patterns.

Table 4. Percentage of mothers breast-feeding on demand and on schedule, by age of child

Country	Group[a]	Age of child							
		0–2 months[b]				3–5 months			
		demand	schedule	other	no. of mothers	demand	schedule	other	no. of mothers
		%	%	%		%	%	%	
Ethiopia	A	43	53	3	30	44	52	4	25
	C	87	13	0	83	79	21	0	78
	R	85	6	9	79	83	7	10	83
Nigeria	A	79	21	0	34	57	43	0	44
	B	79	21	0	47	73	27	0	67
	C	94	6	0	51	96	4	0	75
	R	100	0	0	59	100	0	0	83
Zaire	A	89	11	0	70	84	16	0	75
	C	97	3	0	74	97	3	0	73
	R	92	8	0	74	100	0	0	75
Chile	A	28	72	0	36	8	85	8	26
	C	78	22	0	41	57	41	2	49
	R	86	12	2	43	64	36	0	53
Guatemala	A	46	54	0	74	59	35	6	17
	C	81	19	0	62	77	21	2	47
	R	96	3	1	75	99	0	1	79
India	A	75	7	18	103	62	14	24	80
	B	82	4	14	104	87	4	9	106
	C	97	1	2	99	98	1	2	120
	R	100	0	0	144	99	0	1	146
Philippines	A	86	14	0	35	93	7	0	15
	C	85	15	0	79	89	9	1	76
	R	97	3	0	111	94	6	0	88
Hungary	all	17	82	1	862	21	78	1	666
Sweden	all	56	16	28	111	53	20	27	55

[a] See footnote to Table 1.
[b] 1–2 months in the case of Nigeria, Chile, and Hungary.

Table 5. Frequency of breast-feeding at 0–2 months post partum

Country	Group[a]	No. of feeds by day[b] <4	4–6	7–9	10 or more	average	No. of feeds by night 0	1	2–3	4 or more	average
		%	%	%	%		%	%	%	%	
Ethiopia	A	42	58	0	3.7	7	7	64	21	2.6	
	C	30	60	10	0	4.7	3	7	64	25	2.8
	R	31	44	5	20	5.6	0	7	59	34	3.0
Nigeria	A	20	68	12	0	5.0	3	41	53	3	1.5
	B	17	66	11	6	5.4	2	19	68	11	2.4
	C	6	51	24	20	6.9	2	4	58	36	3.1
	R	0	27	44	29	8.1	0	5	71	24	2.9
Zaire	A	19	48	17	16	6.1	0	6	54	40	2.0
	C	11	45	25	19	6.7	0	7	51	42	2.0
	R	2	57	41	0	6.2	0	0	31	69	3.9
Chile	A	0	92	6	3	5.4	47	39	14	0	0.5
	C	6	71	20	3	5.7	24	21	48	8	1.8
	R	10	58	33	0	5.5	15	34	49	2	1.7
Guatemala	A	8	84	7	1	5.1	16	28	56	0	1.7
	C	19	60	15	6	5.4	2	8	61	29	2.9
	R	6	51	20	23	6.9	1	3	45	51	3.4
India	A	9	50	31	10	5.2	6	22	64	8	2.2
	B	2	63	31	3	6.0	0	8	79	13	3.2
	C	7	30	32	31	7.7	0	8	76	16	2.6
Philippines	A	14	63	14	9	5.7	9	14	63	14	2.3
	C	19	59	14	8	5.2	1	5	52	42	3.2
	R	11	56	17	16	6.2	2	5	31	62	3.6
Hungary	all	8	89	3	0	4.9	67	28	5	0	0.4
Sweden	all	4	93	3	0	5.0	49	46	5	0	0.6

[a] See footnote to Table 1.

[b] "By day" means during mother's waking hours.

In most of the groups studied, feeding patterns did not appear to change markedly between the first and second trimester, mothers tending to maintain for at least 6 months the pattern they developed during the early stages of lactation. The only exceptions to this were in Chile (all groups) and in the Nigerian A group, in which, between the first and second trimester, there was a considerable decline in the proportion feeding on demand. As for patterns after the first 6 months, the numbers involved were too small in most groups to lend themselves to analysis.

Mothers were also asked how many times they breast-fed the baby during the day (defined as "mother's waking hours") and how many times at night. The reliability of the replies to this question, some of which are

Table 6. Percentage of mothers breast-feeding four or more times by day, by age of child*

Country	Group[a]	Age of child (months)					
		0–2[b]	3–5	6–8	9–11	12–14	15–17
		%	%	%	%	%	%
Ethiopia	A	58	46				
	C	70	70	73	77	80	84
	R	69	91	82	80	88	87
Nigeria	A	80	47	55			
	B	83	83	71	71		
	C	94	92	94	96	90	87
	R	100	98	97	98	98	97
Zaire	A	81	81	78	77	82	84
	C	89	86	90	90	74	68
	R	98	97	88	91	94	90
Chile	A	100	84	77			
	C	94	84	67	64		
	R	90	87	76	62	68	46
Guatemala	A	92	88				
	C	81	74	82	61	65	58
	R	94	86	91	87	77	77
India	A	91	71	69	49	39	22
	B	98	83	72	69	64	57
	C	93	96	95	93	90	85
Philippines	A	86	79				
	C	81	92	85	86	81	72
	R	89	88	90	81	91	85
Hungary	all	92	70	29	19		
Sweden	all	96	85	8			

* "By day" means during mother's waking hours.
[a] See footnote to Table 1.
[b] 1–2 months in the case of Nigeria, Chile, and Hungary.

shown in Table 5, is not known, however, and since many mothers tended to feed casually on demand, especially during the night, it may have been difficult for them to have a precise idea of the number of night-feeds given.

The data nevertheless suggest that in almost all the groups (with the exception of the R groups in Nigeria and India) the average number of daytime feeds was 5–7. The daytime frequencies reported were relatively low in all groups in Ethiopia, but high in the C and R groups in Nigeria, the R group in Guatemala, the C group in India, and all groups in Zaire.

Most mothers said that at night they breast-fed 2–3 times, but there were fairly large proportions of mothers in Hungary, Sweden, and Chile (A group) who reported no night-time feeding at all, even at 0–2 months. In the rural groups of Zaire, Guatemala, and the Philippines, most mothers said that they gave 4 or more feeds at night.

Frequent feeding, during both the day and night, was on the whole more common among rural than urban-poor mothers, and in turn more frequent among both these groups than among economically advantaged urban mothers.

Patterns of breast-feeding frequency by age of child are shown in Table 6. The data have been simplified by considering only the proportions of mothers giving 4 or more feeds by day. In Hungary and Sweden, and in all the urban economically advantaged groups except that of Zaire, the percentages fall steeply as the age increases. This is also true of group B in India and groups C and R in Chile. In the remaining groups, the proportions are remarkably constant throughout the age-range covered.

In Hungary and Sweden, about 80 % of mothers discontinued night feeds before the child was 6 months old. In Chile, about 50 % of group-A mothers continued night-feeding until the child was 9 months old (data for higher ages are not available), 1 feed per night being the most common pattern; only around 10 % fed twice or more. In all the other groups studied, breast-feeding at night appears to have been continued by the great majority of mothers; in India, only 17 % of group-A mothers were not feeding at night at 15–17 months post partum; 39 % were still giving 2 or more feeds per night. In the other groups, the percentages of mothers giving 2 or more feeds at night varied from 60 % (India, group B) to 100 % (Ethiopia, group R).

Maternal views on duration of breast-feeding

Mothers were also asked how long they thought breast-feeding should continue before other foods were introduced. As can be seen from Table 7, the answers that were given differed widely in the various groups; in the urban economically advantaged groups of Nigeria, Guatemala, and the Philippines, mothers indicated their preference for short periods of less than 3 months. A similar preference was expressed by many mothers in group R in Ethiopia and in group B in Nigeria. Conversely, in groups C and R in Chile and India there was a tendency to feel that breast-feeding

Table 7. Mothers' views on optimum duration of breast-feeding without supplements

Country	Group[a]	Age to which complete breast-feeding should continue (months)			
		0–2	3–5	6–8	9 or more
		%	%	%	%
Ethiopia	A	7	43	50	0
	C	3	9	80	8
	R	64	21	11	4
Nigeria	A	60	25	12	3
	B	83	12	2	2
	C	36	29	7	27
	R	3	31	35	31
Zaire	A	4	40	50	7
	C	11	31	45	13
	R	31	47	17	5
Chile	A	2	34	49	15
	C	1	17	35	47
	R	1	13	34	52
Guatemala	A	59	36	6	0
	C	15	39	37	10
	R	8	32	40	20
India	A	13	51	30	6
	B	5	33	43	19
	C	1	4	22	73
	R	0	1	9	90
Philippines	A	52	36	10	2
	C	10	56	25	8
	R	1	38	52	9
Hungary	all	5	77	15	2
Sweden	all	0	50	49	1

[a] See footnote to Table 1.

should continue for 9 months or more. With the exception of groups C and R in Nigeria, most of the remaining groups preferred durations of 3–5 months or 6–8 months.

In Zaire, 77 % of mothers in the rural group said they felt breast-feeding should continue until there was a new pregnancy.

Mothers were also asked to say how long breast-feeding should continue altogether. As can be seen in Table 8 only in group A in Guatemala did many mothers (30 %) specify less than 6 months and, in fact, in 9 of the groups studied, all of them urban-poor or rural, there was a clear preference for prolonged breast-feeding. In the remaining groups (including Hungary, Sweden, all the urban economically advantaged and middle-income groups, and the urban-poor groups in Chile, Guatemala, and the Philippines) the preferred durations were 6–8 or 12–14 months.

It is worth noting, however, that the actual duration of breast-feeding was not always consistent with these views and that, notably in Hungary, Sweden, and most of the A groups, many mothers stopped breast-feeding considerably sooner than they considered desirable.

Breast-feeding or bottle-feeding

Mothers were also asked whether they thought breast-feeding or bottle-feeding was better for a child aged 3–6 months, or whether they considered

Table 8. Mothers' views on optimum total length of breast-feeding

Country	Group[a]	Age to which breast-feeding should continue (months)						
		0–2	3–5	6–8	9–11	12–14	15–17	18 or more
		%	%	%	%	%	%	%
Ethiopia	A	0	0	25	6	49	0	19
	C	0	0	1	0	22	0	76
	R	0	0	1	0	9	1	89
Nigeria	A	2	15	50	24	9	0	0
	B	1	2	17	34	36	3	8
	C	0	0	1	2	18	2	77
	R	0	0	0	0	6	1	93
Zaire	A	0	0	5	5	41	11	39
	C	0	0	1	1	22	9	67
Chile	A	1	8	45	11	31	0	4
	C	0	0	13	3	52	1	30
	R	0	1	12	2	52	1	32
Guatemala	A	6	24	57	7	6	0	0
	C	0	1	23	17	49	1	9
	R	0	1	4	6	32	6	51
India	A	0	3	23	16	43	2	13
	B	0	1	6	7	53	1	31
	C	0	0	1	1	5	1	91
	R	0	0	0	0	3	0	97
Philippines	A	4	13	28	4	44	0	7
	C	0	0	8	6	51	6	29
	R	0	0	2	1	43	7	46
Hungary	all	0	5	50	27	17	0	0
Sweden	all	1	4	42	15	34	0	5

[a] See footnote to Table 1.

them equally good. Almost all mothers in group R in Zaire and in groups C and R in India said breast-feeding was better; indeed this was the view of 70% or more of mothers in all groups except in Hungary, where a large majority (74%) of mothers favoured bottle-feeding. The next largest proportion of mothers favouring bottle-feeding (16%) was in the Ethiopian rural group. In the Nigerian and Ethiopian rural groups, more than half the mothers thought that breast and bottle were equally good.

Place of feeding

Mothers were also asked where they preferred to breast-feed: whether at home discreetly; at home without concern for privacy; or anywhere without concern for privacy.

Attitudes differed considerably between countries and groups. Half or more of the mothers in Hungary, Sweden, and all the economically advantaged groups, except in Ethiopia and Zaire, preferred to breast-feed "in privacy", while in most of the rural and urban-poor groups, a majority of mothers said they would breast-feed anywhere without regard to privacy. The same attitude was expressed by nearly 20% of Swedish mothers.

Summary of findings

In Nigeria and Zaire almost all the mothers studied had initiated breast-feeding; in other countries where urban/rural differences were discernible, the pattern was invariably one of a higher prevalence of breast-feeding in the rural group studied. Among the urban economically advantaged (A) groups in the Philippines and Guatemala, a large proportion of the mothers had not breast-fed. The most common reason for not breast-feeding was perceived insufficiency of milk.

Patterns of breast-feeding duration fell into three distinct categories which tended to be associated with the socioeconomic background. In the first of these categories, which included most of the urban economically advantaged groups, the prevalence of breast-feeding at 6 months post partum was never higher than 50%. In the third category, which included most of the rural study groups, 85% of mothers were still breast-feeding at 6 months post partum.

Just as with non-initiation of breast-feeding, the most frequent reason given for stopping breast-feeding, irrespective of child age, was insufficency of milk. Most mothers believed that breast-feeding should continue throughout the first 6 months, although many of them stopped it earlier.

In most groups, the majority of mothers felt that breast-feeding was superior to bottle-feeding.

5. Breast-feeding and reproduction

One of the objectives of the study was to obtain information on the relationship between breast-feeding and reproduction. This section presents data on new pregnancies and the post-partum return of menstruation in relation to breast-feeding patterns, as well as information about contraceptive practices.

Pregnancy at time of interview

At the time of the interview, mothers were asked if they were pregnant; responses were coded "yes", "no", "does not know", or "not stated". Table 9 indicates the proportion of affirmative responses in each group in relation to the overall number of mothers who replied, i.e., excluding those for whom the response was "not stated". Clinical confirmation of pregnancy was available in most cases.

As expected, the prevalence of new pregnancies rose in all groups with the ages of the index children. Although some conceptions did occur during the first 3 months, new pregnancies were generally rare during the first 6 months post partum. During the second 6 months, the highest percentage of reported pregnancies was in the economically advantaged groups of Ethiopia and Nigeria (14% and 13% respectively); the lowest rates during the second 6 months were in the rural groups of Ethiopia, Nigeria, Zaire, and India, among the middle-income and urban-poor groups of Nigeria, and in Sweden. At 12–17 months, pregnancy rates were still lowest among the rural groups; by comparing these data with those in Table 3 it can be seen that the groups with the lowest pregnancy rates are those in which prolonged breast-feeding is almost universal. It will be seen later that the use of contraceptives was low in these particular groups.

At the time of interview it could not be accurately ascertained when mothers who were pregnant again had actually conceived, and it is therefore not possible to say whether they were still breast-feeding at the time of conception. It is possible, however, to identify how many pregnant women were still breast-feeding when interviewed, and also to establish whether pregnancy was said to have occurred without a return of menstruation. The proportion of women becoming pregnant without experiencing a return of menstruation ranged between 1% in Zaire and 11% in Nigeria and Sweden (see Table 10).

Table 9. Percentage of women pregnant at time of interview, by age of child*

Country	Group[a]	Age of index child (months)							
		0–5		6–11		12–17		18 or more	
		%		%		%		%	
Ethiopia	A	3	(87)	14	(90)	32	(59)	26	(46)
	C	1	(181)	6	(172)	15	(128)	21	(91)
	R	0	(165)	0	(171)	5	(136)	15	(105)
Nigeria	A	0	(97)	13	(118)				
	B	0	(119)	1	(139)	17	(142)	30	(149)
	C	0	(126)	0	(168)	2	(165)	7	(150)
	R	0	(142)	0	(163)	1	(169)	4	(166)
Zaire	A	0	(148)	3	(148)	18	(142)	47	(149)
	C	0	(148)	5	(148)	12	(147)	36	(152)
	R	0	(149)	1	(148)	6	(146)	36	(146)
Chile	A	1	(102)	6	(139)				
	C	0	(100)	5	(125)				
	R	0	(102)	9	(119)	9	(129)		
Guatemala	A	1	(278)	6	(235)	16	(55)	13	(15)
	C	1	(147)	8	(147)	15	(152)	20	(133)
	R	0	(160)	3	(179)	10	(146)	30	(98)
India	A	1	(245)	4	(213)	10	(224)	11	(176)
	B	1	(248)	6	(290)	16	(255)	16	(200)
	C	2	(228)	7	(281)	13	(256)	21	(211)
	R	0	(291)	0	(315)	3	(327)	14	(252)
Philippines	A	3	(162)	7	(131)	15	(104)	11	(88)
	C	1	(235)	10	(208)	23	(186)	28	(152)
	R	1	(232)	5	(205)	18	(187)	23	(165)
Hungary	all	0	(3020)	6	(3956)				
Sweden	all	1	(296)	2	(295)				

* Figures in parentheses indicate the numbers of mothers interviewed who stated whether they were pregnant or not.
[a] See footnote to Table 1.

Table 10. Percentages of pregnant women who said they became pregnant without a return of menstruation, by country

Country	Percentage
Ethiopia	8
Nigeria	11
Zaire	4
Chile	1
Guatemala	1
India	7
Philippines	3
Hungary	8
Sweden	11

Table 11. Percentage of pregnant women still breast-feeding index children

Country	Group[a]	Percentage
Ethiopia	A	6
	C	20
	R	30
Nigeria	A	0
	B	1
	C	0
	R	0
Zaire	A	17
	C	16
	R	30
Chile	A	9
	C	0
	R	4
Guatemala	A	0
	C	0
	R	37
India	A	13
	B	30
	C	68
	R	70
Philippines	A	2
	C	16
	R	6
Hungary	all	3
Sweden	all	0

[a] See footnote to Table 1.

Table 11 shows that for several groups pregnancy did not preclude the continuation of breast-feeding. In India, for example, about 70% of all pregnant women in the urban-poor and rural groups were still breast-feeding the index children; in the rural groups of Ethiopia, Zaire, and Guatemala, and also in the B group in India, the proportion was about 30%. In Nigeria, however, hardly any pregnant women were breast-feeding.

Breast-feeding and risk of conception

Any estimation of the risk of conception during, or in the absence of, lactation would require some knowledge of the situation at the time of conception; as indicated earlier, this information was not available. Any

Table 12. Percentage of women pregnant at time of interview, by age of child and according to whether it was being breast-fed (BF) or not breast-fed (NBF)*

Country	Group[a]		Age of index child (months) 0–5	6–11	12–17	18 or more
			%	%	%	%
Ethiopia	C	BF	1 (168)	1 (139)	7 (86)	2 (57)
		NBF	8 (13)	24 (33)	31 (42)	53 (34)
	R	BF	0 (165)	0 (170)	1 (130)	7 (91)
		NBF				71 (14)
Nigeria	C	BF	0 (126)	0 (166)	0 (142)	0 (62)
		NBF			13 (23)	11 (88)
	R	BF	0 (142)	0 (163)	0 (161)	0 (106)
		NBF				12 (60)
Zaire	A	BF	0 (146)	3 (129)	3 (96)	24 (41)
		NBF		5 (19)	50 (46)	56 (108)
	C	BF	0 (148)	1 (141)	4 (125)	8 (78)
		NBF			59 (22)	65 (74)
	R	BF	0 (149)	0 (144)	4 (140)	14 (92)
		NBF				74 (54)
Guatemala	R	BF	0 (153)	1 (164)	6 (125)	16 (58)
		NBF		27 (15)	33 (21)	50 (40)
India	C	BF	2 (219)	6 (266)	9 (234)	16 (174)
		NBF		33 (15)	55 (22)	43 (37)
	R	BF	0 (291)	0 (315)	2 (321)	10 (239)
		NBF				77 (13)

* Groups in which more than about 10% of mothers reported using contraceptives have been excluded. Figures in parentheses indicate the number of mothers interviewed who stated whether they were pregnant or not.
[a] See footnote to Table 1.

such calculation should also take into account factors other than lactation that diminish or eliminate the risk of conception, e.g., the use of contraceptives, abstinence, or sterilization. Table 12 shows, for some groups, the percentage of women who were pregnant at the time of interview and whether they were breast-feeding; but the data do not, of course, reveal the proportion breast-feeding at the time of conception.

As can be seen from Fig. 4, which illustrates the data presented in Table 12, in all groups and at all ages of the index children the proportion of women who were pregnant was considerably lower among those who were currently breast-feeding than among those who were not.

It is important to note, however, that the differences in the percentage of pregnancies between the breast-feeding and non-breast-feeding categories must be considerably greater than the differences in risk of conception because, among women who were not breast-feeding when interviewed, the group who were pregnant included some who were breast-feeding at the time of conception but had stopped doing so between the time of

Fig. 4. Percentage of women pregnant, by breast-feeding status, 12–17 months post partum*

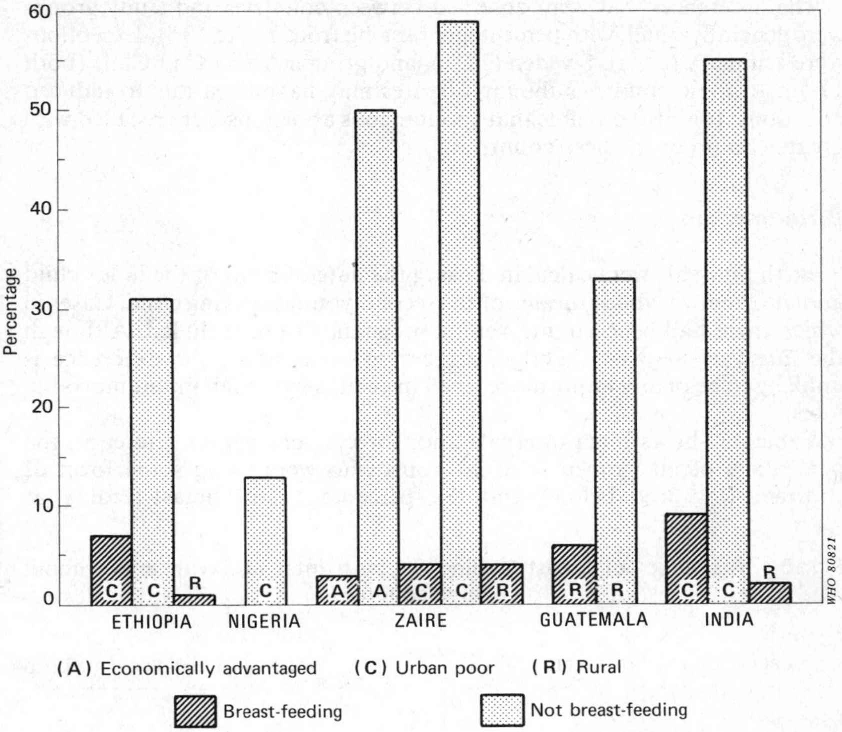

Source: Table 12.
*Groups in which more than 10% of mothers reported using contraceptives have been excluded.

conception and the interview. Also, abstention from intercourse during the period of lactation in some groups may have reinforced the natural reduction of fertility in breast-feeding mothers; this was felt to be an important factor in Nigeria, for example.

For these reasons, the differences in pregnancy rates between breast-feeding mothers and those not breast-feeding, as shown in Table 12 and in Fig. 4, exaggerate (probably considerably) the relative risk of conception in these two categories.

Intervening pregnancies

Each mother was also asked whether she had been pregnant, or had given birth to another child, between the index child and the previous living child. While the information obtained by this question does not indicate the outcome of intervening pregnancies, it does provide an insight into pregnancies that did not result in a child who was still alive at the time of the interview.

The differences that were observed between countries and study groups were generally small, with percentages ranging from 7 % to 13 %. Exceptions were Hungary (27 %), Sweden (20 %), and groups A and C in Chile (both 17 %). In these countries the high figures may have been due to induced abortions. It is also possible that spontaneous abortions were recalled with greater accuracy in these countries.

Birth intervals

Birth intervals were calculated using the date of birth of the index child and information about the age of the second youngest living child. Cases in which there had been an intervening pregnancy were excluded. Although the intervals may be slightly exaggerated as a result, the difference is unlikely to be of any importance, even in groups with high infant mortality rates.

Table 13 shows birth intervals and, for convenience of reference, the percentage of all women in each group who were using some form of contraception (see below) and the percentage still breast-feeding at

Fig. 5. The effect of breast-feeding on birth intervals, with and without contraception

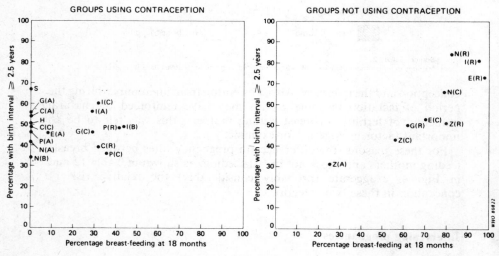

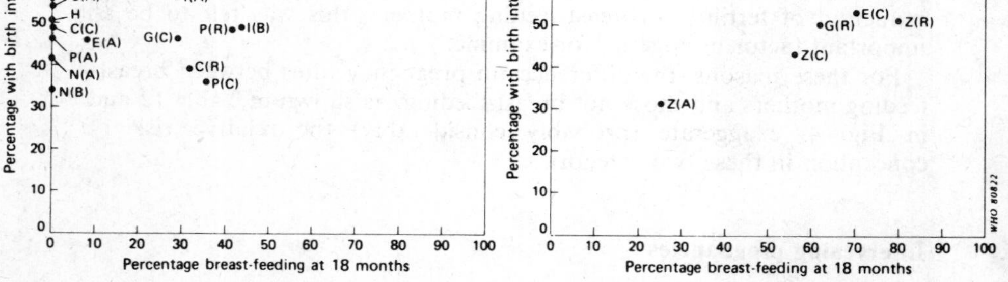

E:Ethiopia N:Nigeria Z:Zaire C:Chile G:Guatemala I:India H:Hungary S:Sweden

(A) Economically advantaged (B) Urban middle income (C) Urban poor (R) Rural

Source: Table 13.

Table 13. Percentages of women for whom the interval between the birth of the index child and that of the second youngest living child was up to 2.5 years or more than 2.5 years, of those using some form of contraception, and of those breast-feeding at 18 months post partum

Country	Group[a]	Percentage for whom birth interval was		Percentage	
		up to 2.5 years[b]	more than 2.5 years[b]	using contraception	breast-feeding at 18 months post partum
Ethiopia	A	54	46	56	8
	C	47	53	4	70
	R	27	73	0	97
Nigeria	A	59	41	30	0
	B	66	34	16	0
	C	34	66	0	79
	R	16	84	0	82
Zaire	A	69	31	10	25
	C	57	43	3	56
	R	49	51	0	80
Chile	A	46	54	71	0
	C	51	49	57	0
	R	61	39	59	32
Guatemala	A	45	55	87	0
	C	54	46	34	29
	R	55	50	4	61
India	A	44	56	67	29
	B	51	49	51	44
	C	40	60	11	31
	R	18	82	4	95
Philippines	A	53	47	75	0
	C	64	36	46	35
	R	51	49	34	42
Hungary	all	49	51	77	0
Sweden	all	33	67	95	0

[a] See footnote to Table 1.
[b] Not including women having had intervening pregnancies.

18 months post partum. From Fig. 5, which shows the data in a graphic form and separates those groups in which more than 10 % of mothers were using contraception, it is evident that, in the absence of contraception, prolonged breast-feeding is associated with longer birth intervals. It is interesting to note that, in groups in which more than 10 % of women were using contraception, the percentage with long birth intervals is lower than in those in which the majority of mothers breast-fed for at least 18 months.

Use of contraception

Because the question was optional, not all women were asked about family planning. Nevertheless, in practice the question was put to at least 80 % of women in all the groups and in many it was posed to all women.

As can be seen from Table 14, the proportion of mothers using contraception varied widely, ranging from 95 % in Sweden to very few in most rural groups, except in Chile and the Philippines. In all countries, there was a decreasing gradient from group A to group B and group R; in groups in which contraception was not widely practised, there was little to indicate that the extent of contraceptive use increased with time (see also Annex 1, Table A2).

The types of contraceptive method used are given in Table 14, which shows that there are considerable differences between countries, whereas the differences between groups within countries are much less marked. Condoms were common in Sweden and in the A and B groups in Nigeria and India. Intrauterine devices were very common in Chile and quite common in the A and C groups in Ethiopia. Oral contraceptives were used by 60 % of mothers in Hungary, but by only 30 % of mothers in Sweden. In the developing countries in the study, oral contraceptives were used fairly commonly in groups A and C in Ethiopia, group A in Zaire, and all groups in Chile, Guatemala, and the Philippines, but rather rarely in all the Indian groups. The rhythm method was common in group A in Ethiopia, groups A and C in Zaire, and the A groups in Guatemala and the Philippines. Coitus interruptus was a commonly used method in groups C and R in the Philippines, and in Hungary. In India, Guatemala, and the Philippines, the proportions of mothers mentioning other methods were high; these methods include surgical sterilization (male or female), injectable contraceptives, and vaginal tablets. There was little evidence that diaphragms or foam were widely used in any country.

Among mothers using oral contraception, a large majority began to use them in the first 3 months post partum. In the countries where there were a large number of oral contraceptive users, between 43 % and 64 % began to use them in the first 2 months, and between 65 % and 76 % in the first 3 months. Between 18 % and 40 % of users started taking them while still breast-feeding, up to 23 % taking them before the breast-fed baby was 3 months old.

Table 14. Number and percentage of mothers using contraception and their percentage distribution by type of contraception*

Country	Group[a]	Users		Percentage distribution of users by type of contraception used							
		no.	as percentage of those questioned	condom	IUD	diaphragm	oral	foam	rhythm	coitus interruptus	other
Ethiopia	A	151	56	3	26	1	34	0	31	4	2
	C	22	4	0	23	5	59	0	5	0	9
	R	2	0								
Nigeria	A	71	30	31	25	6	8	7	15	3	4
	B	92	16	18	13	5	17	7	8	4	24
	C	1	0								
	R	1	0								
Zaire	A	59	10	3	10	0	19	2	47	0	14
	C	19	3	5	5	0	5	8	79	0	0
	R	1	0								
Chile	A	202	71	1	50	1	26	3	8	0	0
	C	160	57	0	67	1	18	1	2	0	13
	R	245	59	3	64	1	18	0	0	0	14
Guatemala	A	414	87	10	17	1	35	3	22	0	15
	C	157	34	4	17	3	45	1	1	1	32
	R	20	4	0	10	0	55	0	5	0	30
India	A	502	67	49	8	0	8	1	8	1	25
	B	418	51	31	5	0	3	0	2	0	57
	C	90	11	10	4	0	1	0	1	0	83
	R	47	4	0	0	0	0	0	0	0	100
Philippines	A	331	75	17	2	0	27	2	38	8	23
	C	308	46	9	16	0	26	0	18	31	14
	R	242	34	7	2	0	24	0	16	46	7
Hungary	all	6028	77	6	11	1	60	1	3	17	1
Sweden	all	477	95	49	15	2	30	7	1	5	0

* Those questioned included pregnant women; the percentage distribution by type of contraception may sometimes add up to more than 100 as multiple answers were possible.
[a] See footnote to Table 1.

Return of menstruation

An analysis of the percentages of women who were menstruating again at various ages post partum shows that, at 6 months, 90% or more of mothers in Hungary and in the A groups in Ethiopia, Guatemala, and the Philippines had experienced a return of menstruation. In Sweden and the A groups of Nigeria and India, and in all groups in Chile, 70–80 % of mothers were menstruating at 6 months post partum; in all rural groups, however, especially in Zaire and India, the proportion of mothers menstruating again was particularly low.

By 12 months post partum, nearly all the mothers studied in Hungary, Sweden, and in all the A groups except that of Zaire reported a return of menstruation. But in the C and R groups of Ethiopia, Nigeria, and India and in the R group of Zaire the proportion menstruating again at 12 months was never higher than 40%.

The remaining groups fall into an intermediate range; at 18 months post partum, only about 50% of women in the rural groups of Ethiopia, Nigeria, and India had experienced a return of menstruation.

Within the countries, then, there was a marked gradient, the return of menstruation occurring latest in the R groups and earliest in the A and B groups.

Fig 6 shows the percentages of women with return of menstruation, grouped according to the three categories I, II, and III that have already been used to distinguish breast-feeding patterns (see page 33 and Fig. 3). It shows that this classification may very well be used to distinguish patterns of the return of menstruation also. As was the case in Fig. 3, the scatter is least in Category I (in which breast-feeding diminished rapidly) and greatest in Category III (in which breast-feeding was prolonged).

An analysis of percentages of menstruating women at various times post partum, with the corresponding percentages of breast-feeding women considered as an independent variable, shows that 85% of the total variability between countries and groups in respect of return of menstruation can be attributed to differences in breast-feeding behaviour.[1]

Table 15 shows the percentages of women who had experienced a return of menstruation, by various child ages, and whether they were breast-feeding (fully or partially) or not. It is of interest that, among those not breast-feeding at the time of the interview, the percentages with returned menstruation are remarkably uniform in all groups. By contrast, the percentages among women who were breast-feeding vary widely from group to group. The data show that breast-feeding is associated with a considerable delay in the return of menstruation, but that the differences between breast-feeding and non-breast-feeding mothers gradually diminish or disappear with time.

---

[1] BILLEWICZ, W. Z. The timing of post-partum menstruation and breast feeding: a simple formula. *Journal of biosocial science*, **11**; 141–151 (1979).

Fig. 6. Percentage of mothers with return of menstruation, by age of child and population group (three categories)

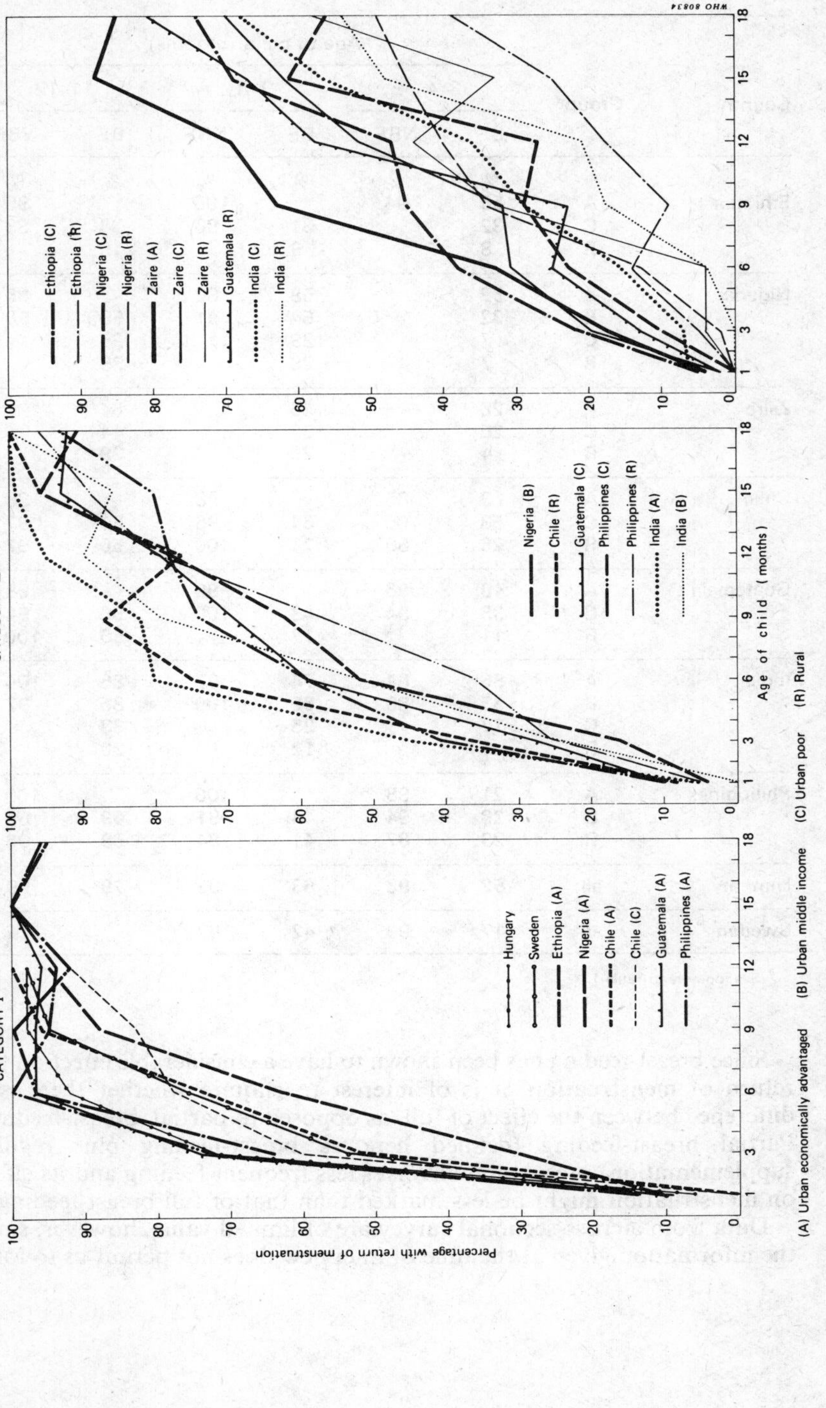

Table 15. Percentage of women with return of menstruation by age of child and whether it was being breast-fed (BF) or not breast-fed (NBF)

Country	Group[a]	Age of child (months)					
		3–4		7–8		11–12	
		BF	NBF	BF	NBF	BF	NBF
		%	%	%	%	%	%
Ethiopia	A	56	94		100		95
	C	32		31	90	38	83
	R	8		9		16	
Nigeria	A	52		58	82		95
	B	32		54	91	50	90
	C	7		29		25	
	R	7		28		39	
Zaire	A	26		46		64	
	C	25		32		44	
	R	4		20		39	
Chile	A	23	85		98		98
	C	53	100	64	96	69	97
	R	26	80	71	100	56	97
Guatemala	A	40	96		99		98
	C	35	94	43	100	50	94
	R	11		17		50	100
India	A	56	84	74	97	86	100
	B	33	80	62	100	85	97
	C	17		25		33	
	R	1		12		20	
Philippines	A	21	98		100		100
	C	28	94	44	91	69	88
	R	23	87	41	94	69	96
Hungary	all	52	93	63	98	79	99
Sweden	all	17	93	42	97		

[a] See footnote to Table 1.

Since breast-feeding has been shown to have a considerable effect on the return of menstruation, it is of interest to enquire whether there is a difference between the effect of full, as opposed to partial, breast-feeding. Partial breast-feeding (defined here as breast-feeding plus regular supplementation) presumably involves less frequent feeding and its effect on menstruation might be less marked than that of full breast-feeding.

Data from a cross-sectional survey are of limited value, however, since the information given at the time of interview does not permit us to infer with any certainty that menstruation had returned while the mother was fully or partially breast-feeding.

A further difficulty is that in most groups, during the immediate post-partum period, the great majority of breast-fed babies were fully breast-fed; later on, this situation reversed itself so that most babies were receiving regular supplements. As a result, sufficient numbers of fully breast-fed and regularly supplemented children of the same age are found in only a few groups.

Information from India (groups B and C), the Philippines (all groups), Chile (groups A and C), Zaire (group C), and Ethiopia (group A) suggests that menstruation tends to return sooner when there is partial breast-feeding then when there is full breast-feeding. In Hungary, where numbers were large, comparisons indicated no consistent difference. The same was true of the C and R groups in Ethiopia and the R groups in Zaire and Chile, although numbers were much smaller in these groups than in Hungary.

Because partial breast-feeding, defined with reference to the use of regular (daily) supplements, could imply considerably different frequencies of suckling, breast-feeding frequency was also examined in relation to menstruation. As noted above, however, it should be borne in mind that mothers in some groups may not have accurately reported the number of times they breast-fed their babies.

Table 16 summarizes, as examples of "positive" findings, the data for the urban-poor and rural groups in Guatemala and for Hungary. Frequency-of-suckling categories of "up to 4 times" and "5 times or more" by day (mothers' waking hours) were adopted. The percentages of women in whom menstruation had returned were consistently higher, irrespective of post-partum interval, among the women who suckled least frequently.

Table 16. Percentage of breast-feeding women with return of menstruation, by age of child and frequency of suckling, Guatemala and Hungary*

Country	Frequency of suckling by day[a]	Age of child (months)		
		1–4	5–8	9–12
Guatemala[b]	up to 4 times	22 (59)	42 (53)	53 (74)
	5 times or more	11 (115)	23 (124)	36 (90)
Hungary	up to 4 times	49 (308)	68 (435)	
	5 times or more	26 (1 006)	51 (79)	

* Figures in parentheses indicate numbers of breast-feeding women interviewed.
[a] "By day" means during mother's waking hours.
[b] Urban poor (C) and rural (R) groups.

Among mothers who never breast-fed, it was possible to estimate frequency of returned menstruation by using retrospective data and amalgamating groups in which there were data on mothers. About 90% of these mothers were menstruating at 4 months post partum. In the absence of breast-feeding, there was a slight delay in groups C and R compared with groups A and B.

Summary of findings

New pregnancies were rare in the first 6 months post partum. Their incidence throughout the first year was consistently lowest among the rural groups studied. Between 1 % and 11 % of the mothers who were found to be pregnant since giving birth to the index children did not first experience a return of menstruation.

On the whole there were few differences between countries with respect to the incidence of intervening pregnancies not resulting in a child who was still alive at the time of the study. The differences that did emerge in Hungary, Sweden, and Chile may have been due to a greater recall of spontaneous abortions. Birth intervals were generally longest in the rural groups and longer in the urban-poor than higher-income groups. In groups where few or no women used contraception, the length of the birth interval was closely related to the length of breast-feeding.

The highest utilization of contraceptive methods (other than abstinence) was found in Sweden. Family planning appears to have made little inroad in the rural areas of the other countries and even in some urban-poor communities the prevalence of family planning was low. Contraceptive use decreased with the socioeconomic status of the community. Methods varied considerably, but oral contraception appeared to be the most popular, and the diaphragm and foam the least commonly used, of all methods.

Post-partum amenorrhea was more prolonged in rural populations and appeared to follow the pattern of breast-feeding fairly closely. Some of the data also suggest that, in certain groups, full as opposed to partial breast-feeding lends itself to prolongation of amenorrhea. There was also a tendency in some groups for frequent suckling to be associated with delayed return of menstruation.

6. Family characteristics, maternal health, health care practices, and breast-feeding

The background of the parents can be expected to influence patterns of infant care and feeding. Similarly, the situation with regard to health services and working conditions during the processes of pregnancy and delivery and the early postnatal period may play an important part. This chapter presents a summary of the information obtained on these factors and their association with patterns of breast-feeding in the groups studied (see also Annex 1, Table A3).

Age, parity, and breast-feeding

Maternal age and parity are highly correlated and, in many cases, their separate effects on breast-feeding patterns are difficult to distinguish. In order to maximize numbers and thus facilitate analysis, recall information about the duration of breast-feeding has been used, together with point-prevalence data. When age and parity were considered simultaneously, trends by age within parity groups and trends by parity within age groups appeared only in Sweden, where, at 3 months post partum, breast-feeding was more common among mothers with first babies and among older mothers.

At 12 months, no associations were found with either maternal age or parity, except, perhaps, in the A and B groups in India, in which there was some indication that women of high parity were more likely to breast-feed.

Education and occupation of the mother

Maternal educational and occupational characteristics are highly correlated, and their separate effects on breast-feeding are difficult to distinguish. The fact that the population groups studied were selected in a manner that necessarily tended to yield homogeneous occupational and educational categories also obscures possible differences. For the purposes of the study, "occupation" was taken to include work which the mother might have performed at some previous time, or prior to pregnancy, even though she was not gainfully employed at the time of the survey.

Table 17. Percentage of mothers breast-feeding index children, by maternal education and age of child, in selected groups

Country	Group[a]	Maternal education	Age of child (months) 0–2	3–5	6–8
			%	%	%
India	A	secondary	96 (47)	74 (43)	63 (51)
		university	84 (69)	56 (85)	38 (65)
India	B	primary	96 (24)	97 (31)	90 (29)
		secondary	91 (89)	73 (104)	72 (108)
Philippines	C	primary	74 (50)	71 (68)	57 (53)
		secondary	66 (65)	53 (53)	49 (61)
Philippines	R	primary	93 (94)	81 (88)	87 (84)
		secondary	86 (28)	77 (22)	70 (30)
Sweden	all	primary	58 (50)	18 (38)	18 (40)
		secondary	79 (78)	40 (89)	24 (85)
		university	95 (21)	62 (21)	38 (24)

* Groups in which no association was found are omitted. In the A and B groups in India and in Sweden, the association is significant. Figures in parentheses indicate numbers of mothers in each of the relevant categories.
[a] See footnote to Table 1.

Table 17, in which only educational categories are considered, shows that there was a tendency for the prevalence of breast-feeding in Sweden, at all child ages, to increase with the mother's educational status. Among the urban poor and rural groups in the Philippines, on the other hand, and among the A and B groups in India, the trends observed are in the opposite direction. In all other groups in which it was possible to investigate this point, trends by education were absent.

Mothers' past experience with breast-feeding

Mothers were also asked about any previous experience with breast-feeding, in particular how long they had completely breast-fed (i.e., breast-fed without supplementation) their second-youngest children. Three possible responses were allowed for: ". . . months", "does not recall", or "not applicable". Because "not applicable" appears to have been interpreted by interviewers in various ways (some applied it to cases in which a previous child was not breast-fed at all, as well as to primaparae), "not applicable" responses have been excluded from Table 18.

Present breast-feeding behaviour appears to have been related to whether, and for how long, a mother had breast-fed her previous child. As

Table 18. Percentage of mothers breast-feeding index children, according to whether their second-youngest children were completely breast-fed for less or more than 1 month*

Country	Group[a]	Duration of breast-feeding of second-youngest child	
		less than 1 month	1 month or more
		%	%
Ethiopia	A	58 (19)	95 (99)
Chile	A	88 (49)	98 (118)
	C	88 (25)	100 (146)
	R	100 (32)	98 (259)
Guatemala	A	69 (91)	97 (75)
	C	77 (22)	96 (280)
	R	100 (39)	99 (412)
Philippines	A	52 (93)	85 (198)
	C	70 (27)	96 (423)
	R	91 (69)	96 (502)
India	A	76 (49)	98 (455)
	B	73 (33)	98 (585)
	C	91 (11)	99 (548)
Hungary	all	89 (602)	66 (3690)
Sweden	all	83 (90)	94 (218)

* Figures in parentheses indicate numbers of mothers in each of the relevant categories.
[a] See footnote to Table 1.

the data in Table 18 show, in the A and C groups and in Hungary and Sweden, a mother who had breast-fed her previous child for more than 1 month was more inclined to breast-feed the index child, and vice versa. In the R groups, the two factors seemed to be unrelated. In India, a considerable proportion of mothers did not answer the question at all.

Mothers were also asked whether they themselves had been breast-fed, but since 80 % or more in all groups answered affirmatively, no analysis of the effects on their current breast-feeding behaviour was undertaken.

Length of residence

The possible influence of migration on infant-feeding practices was considered, using "less than 3 years" or "3 years and over" as the measurement of length of residence. No significant association with the prevalence of breast-feeding emerged.

Type of family

The amount of social support available to mothers with young children is likely to vary with family circumstances, and mothers were therefore asked whether the families in which they lived were nuclear, extended, or "other".

The only situation in which an association emerged between the prevalence of breast-feeding and family type was in Guatemala among the urban economically advantaged (A) group:[1]

	Nuclear families	*Extended families*
Mother breast-feeding at 0–2 months	46% (122)	65% (31)
Mother breast-feeding at 3–5 months	9% (93)	27% (33)

The differences are statistically significant.

As far as the background characteristics of husbands are concerned, no independent relationships were found between the prevalence of breast-feeding, or breast-feeding behaviour, and a husband's age, education, occupation, employment status, or whether he was currently residing with the wife.

Prenatal care

Visits to prenatal clinics can be important from the point of view of preparing the mother for child care and feeding, and mothers were therefore asked whether they had attended a prenatal clinic and, if so, how often. Table 19 summarizes the responses.

As might be expected from the nature of the groups selected for study, there were large differences between them with respect to the use of prenatal services. For example, in Sweden, Hungary, and all the economically advantaged groups, most women had received prenatal care and most mothers had paid more than 3 visits to prenatal services. In the rural groups of Ethiopia and India, the proportions of mothers who had not received prenatal care were as high as 88% and 56% respectively. Fewer than one-quarter of all mothers in the C and R groups of Zaire attended prenatal clinics more than 3 times.

A comparison of these data with those in Table 2 suggests that, for the most part, the groups with the highest provision (or utilization) of prenatal care had the lowest prevalence and shortest durations of breast-feeding. In Ethiopia and India, where there was a suggestion of some variation within groups, breast-feeding tended to be less common among those who had received the most prenatal care. Although this correlation is probably spurious and due to selection factors inherent in the samples, the data do

[1] Figures in parentheses indicate numbers of families in the relevant categories.

not provide any clear evidence that prenatal care played a positive part in the promotion of breast-feeding among the groups that were studied.

Table 19. Percentage of mothers who had attended or not attended prenatal clinics, by number of visits

Country	Group[a]	No. of visits			
		none	1–3	4–9	10 or more
		%	%	%	%
Ethiopia	A	1	5	30	63
	C	29	16	41	13
	R	88	10	2	0
Nigeria	A	0	0	18	81
	B	2	1	39	58
	C	8	5	64	23
	R	15	3	26	56
Zaire	A	4	53	41	1
	C	12	60	26	1
	R	13	63	23	1
Chile	A	0	1	69	30
	C	5	6	72	17
	R	9	7	70	13
Guatemala	A	0	1	13	86
	C	28	16	51	5
	R	34	29	35	2
India	A	3	4	34	61
	B	7	35	43	4
	C	46	27	24	2
	R	56	33	10	0
Philippines	A	1	4	34	61
	C	17	35	43	4
	R	11	39	40	10
Hungary	all	0	1	50	49
Sweden	all	0	1	6	93

[a] See footnote to Table 1.

Health during pregnancy

Because health records for mothers in many of the study groups were likely to be unavailable, mothers were asked directly about their state of health during pregnancy. The data thus represent the opinions of mothers which it was not possible to check.

The majority of mothers in all groups said they had been healthy. Only in the R group in Ethiopia and the C group in Chile, where respectively 18%

and 14 % of the respondents said they had been very ill, did the proportion ever rise above 10 %. In groups where prenatal care was uncommon, or the number of prenatal visits few, it is possible that there was some association between available care and maternal health, but this could not be pursued in the study because of the small numbers involved.

As far as the possible effects of maternal health during pregnancy are concerned, there was no evidence that it was in any way associated with the prevalence and duration of breast-feeding.

Paid employment during pregnancy

In order to determine whether employment status during pregnancy might have influenced breast-feeding, mothers were asked (*a*) if they had

Table 20. Percentage of all mothers in paid employment during pregnancy and percentage of working mothers given paid leave post partum

Country	Group[a]	Percentage of all mothers working	Percentage of working mothers with paid leave
Ethiopia	A	73	98
	C	23	91
	R	0	
Nigeria	A	83	96
	B	56	96
	C	0	
	R	0	
Zaire	A	8	94
	C	0	
	R	0	
Chile	A	32	83
	C	16	62
	R	5	68
Guatemala	A	33	61
	C	19	25
	R	12	3
India	A	6	91
	B	8	95
	C	7	25
	R	56	0
Philippines	A	33	71
	C	9	24
	R	5	21
Hungary	all	88	100
Sweden	all	72	100

[a] See footnote to Table 1.

been in paid employment during pregnancy; (*b*) if they had been given paid leave after delivery and, if so, for how long; and also (*c*) if they had been working (full-time or part-time) during the month when the interview took place.

As can be seen from Table 20, in Hungary, Sweden, the Ethiopian A group, the Nigerian A and B groups, and the Indian R group, most mothers were gainfully employed during pregnancy, as were about one-third of the mothers in the A groups of Chile, Guatemala, and the Philippines. In the remaining groups, it was relatively uncommon for mothers to be in paid employment, although this does not necessarily mean that mothers did only domestic work; in the rural groups, for example, it is probable that they were also engaged in agricultural work that did not involve financial remuneration.

In Hungary, Sweden, Ethiopia, and Nigeria, and among the economically advantaged of Zaire, nearly all those who had been in paid employment (more than 90%) took paid post-partum leave. In Chile, where all working women were apparently entitled to paid leave, only some 60–80% said they received it, but this may have reflected the fact that the payments were made in two parts and many mothers had not received a payment before they were interviewed. In Guatemala, eligibility for paid leave was limited to those in government service and in large industries, which explains the low proportions found in the urban-poor and rural groups. The percentages of women given paid leave in the Philippine C and R groups were also low, because the labour code covered only those in government work and private industry and not those in agricultural work, cottage industries, etc. Similarly, in India paid leave was available only to women in government posts and in large industries, which again probably explains the high percentages in groups A and B, and the low percentages in groups C and R (Table 20).

Place of delivery and stay in hospital

Almost all mothers in Hungary and Sweden and in the economically advantaged and middle-income groups in the other countries studied reported the place of delivery as a hospital or a health centre. Among rural mothers (R groups), hospital deliveries ranged from 86% in Chile to less than 15% in Ethiopia, Guatemala, the Philippines, and India (Table 21).

Among mothers delivered at home, a considerable proportion were unassisted or were delivered by unskilled attendants; this was particularly so among the urban-poor and rural groups of Ethiopia, Nigeria, and Zaire. In the Philippines, deliveries by a trained attendant predominated, but in other countries traditional birth attendants were the most common source of assistance, especially in rural areas.

Among those delivered in hospital in Hungary, and in the urban economically advantaged, middle-income, and rural groups of India, about half of all mothers were confined for 7 days or more. This was also the case in Zaire among the rural group but not among urban mothers

Table 21. Place of delivery and type of attendant at delivery*

Country	Group[a]	Percentage delivered at home with trained attendant	at home with traditional birth attendant	at home with unskilled attendant alone	in institution
Ethiopia	A	1	1	1	97
	C	2	22	24	52
	R	1	16	82	1
Nigeria	A	0	0	0	100
	B	0	3	1	96
	C	1	11	17	72
	R	1	20	34	46
Zaire	A	1	12	11	76
	C	1	26	34	39
	R	4	33	16	57
Chile	A	0	0	0	100
	C	0	0	2	98
	R	0	2	11	86
Guatemala	A	0	0	0	100
	C	7	2	2	89
	R	3	79	4	13
India	A	4	1	0	96
	B	5	6	0	89
	C	6	46	2	46
	R	2	77	11	9
Philippines	A	3	0	0	97
	C	27	15	1	58
	R	66	26	0	8
Hungary	all	0	0	0	100
Sweden	all	0	0	0	100

* The category "delivered in other place than home or institution" was very small in all groups and is excluded. Percentages may not add up to 100, owing to rounding.

[a] See footnote to Table 1.

(A and C groups), who tended to stay in hospital for 3 days or less. In the urban areas of Zaire, hospital confinement involved some payment, which may have encouraged early discharge; in the rural areas, many of the hospital and clinics are run by foreign organizations and there is a pattern of post-partum supervision over 6–7 days, even in uncomplicated cases. In general most other mothers reported a stay in hospital of 3 days or less. Sweden was an exception, falling between the two extremes (see Table 22).

Although the number of mothers involved was very small, in the urban-poor and rural groups in Guatemala and in the rural group in the

Table 22. Length of stay in institution post partum*

Country	Group[a]	Length of stay (in days) less than 4	4 to 6	7 or more
		%	%	%
Ethiopia	A	51	29	20
	C	71	22	7
Nigeria	A	53	31	16
	B	68	26	6
	C	84	13	3
	R	81	18	1
Zaire	A	60	25	15
	C	74	15	11
	R	2	39	59
Chile	A	60	37	3
	C	45	43	12
	R	46	37	17
Guatemala	A	48	42	10
	C	77	14	9
	R	86	9	5
India	A	16	34	50
	B	31	23	46
	C	61	17	22
Philippines	A	41	38	21
	C	75	16	9
Hungary	all	3	39	58[b]
Sweden	all	1	76	23

* The percentages are based on the numbers of mothers delivered in hospital.

[a] See footnote to Table 1.
[b] 6 days or more.

Philippines, there was a clear tendency for breast-feeding to be more common among mothers who were delivered at home than among those delivered in hospital. In the case of the urban-poor groups in Ethiopia and the Philippines, where the numbers of mothers involved were larger, there was a significantly higher prevalence of breast-feeding following home delivery. In some groups, notably the urban-poor and rural groups in the Philippines, the proportion of mothers who never breast-fed was higher among those who were delivered in hospital.

Although in Sweden there was a slight tendency for the prevalence of breast-feeding to be lower among mothers whose stays in hospital were relatively short, in general there was no association in other countries between the length of confinement and the prevalence of breast-feeding.

Rooming-in

Mothers who were delivered in hospitals or maternity centres were asked if the baby had been kept in the same room with them; Table 23 shows the relevant percentages. As can be seen there were wide differences between countries and study groups. While "rooming-in" was nearly universal in Nigeria, India, and the urban groups in Zaire, and practised in over 80% of group A cases in Ethiopia, and the C and R groups in Chile, the percentage of babies kept with the mothers in Hungary, the R group in Zaire, all groups in Guatemala, and groups A and R in the Philippines was low.

Table 23. Percentage of babies delivered in institutions who were kept in the same room as the mother

Country	Group[a]				
	A	B	C	R	all
	%	%	%	%	%
Ethiopia	84		68	[b]	
Nigeria	92	93	98	98	
Zaire	91		94	2	
Chile	15		82	85	
Guatemala	2		5	9	
India	97	98	98	99	
Philippines	2		18	6	
Hungary					1
Sweden					31

[a] See footnote to Table 1.
[b] 3 out of 4 cases.

Differences in "rooming-in" practices arise not only from hospital routines but also from different medical attitudes to the desirability of keeping mother and baby together. In some instances, however, (e.g., in the Philippines) the low frequency of "rooming-in" also reflected a shortage of physical facilities designed for the purpose.

Table 24. Percentage of mothers breast-feeding, by age of child, according to whether the baby was kept in the same room as the mother after delivery or in a separate room, Chile and Sweden

Country and group[a]	Room	Age of child (months)					
		0–2		3–5		6–8	
Chile: A	same	88	(8)	40	(15)	27	(11)
	separate	69	(42)	34	(58)	17	(64)
C and R	same	87	(79)	74	(110)	50	(112)
	separate	69	(13)	42	(24)	31	(29)
Sweden	same	80	(54)	46	(52)	27	(52)
	separate	72	(95)	33	(96)	23	(97)

* Groups in which numbers were low or no association was apparent are excluded. Figures in parentheses indicate the numbers of mothers interviewed.
[a] See footnote to Table 1.

A useful analysis of the relationship of "rooming-in" to subsequent breast-feeding performance was feasible only in the case of Chile and Sweden, where there were reasonable numbers both of babies kept with the mother and of babies kept separate from the mother. Table 24 suggests that, in these two countries, "rooming-in" favoured breast-feeding; but the differences were not statistically significant. A similar tendency was seen in the data group C in the Philippines, but the number of mothers involved was small. It is worth noting, however, that in the rural group in Zaire prolonged breast-feeding was universal, although there was virtually no "rooming-in".

Free gifts of milk or feeding-bottles in health facilities

Mothers delivered in hospital were asked whether they had received free milk samples or a free feeding-bottle while in hospital. No responses were obtained from mothers in Hungary, and the practice of providing such gifts was either non-existent or rare in Sweden, Zaire, and India, and among the urban-poor and rural groups in Chile.

As shown in Table 25, data for the remaining countries indicate that, on the whole, more than 10 % of all mothers who were delivered in hospital in the A and B groups in Nigeria, the C group in Guatemala, and the A and R groups in the Philippines were given free milk samples. It is particularly noteworthy that in the Philippines over 27 % of mothers in the economically advantaged group and 41 % of the mothers in the rural group were given free gifts of milk.

Table 25. Percentage of mothers delivered in hospital who received free gifts of milk or feeding-bottles*

Country	Group[a]	No. of mothers	Percentage receiving	
			free milk	free bottles
Ethiopia	A	284	8	6
	C	305	7	5
Nigeria	A	234	24	10
	B	549	16	1
	C	451	10	1
	R	307	5	3
Chile	A	295	6	0
Guatemala	A	591	5	2
	C	527	19	13
	R	79	5	4
Philippines	A	480	27	4
	C	455	9	2
	R	63	41	3

* Gifts were rare in groups other than those given here.
[a] See footnote to Table 1.

In Guatemala, among the urban-poor group, the prevalence of breast-feeding at 0–2 and 3–5 months post partum was lower among mothers who had been given such gifts; the numbers, however, were too low for the differences to be statistically significant. In the other groups there was no evidence of a consistent trend, although in the Philippines a large proportion of mothers in the A group were given free milk samples and this may have been related to the high percentage of mothers who did not breast-feed. On the other hand, more than 40 % of the R-group mothers delivered in hospital were given free milk, and a comparison with other hospitalized mothers in the same group suggests that this did not affect the prevalence of breast-feeding.

The provision of free bottles was less common: the highest percentages were observed in Nigeria, where about 10 % of mothers in group A reported having been given a bottle, and in Guatemala, where 13 % of mothers in group C were given them.

Timing of first breast-feed

Mothers were asked whether the baby was given the breast immediately (i.e., within the first 12 hours) after birth, or later. Because of the difficulty

Table 26. Percentage of mothers who put the child to the breast within 12 hours of delivery, by place of delivery

Country	Place of delivery	Group[a]				
		A	B	C	R	all
		%	%	%	%	
Ethiopia	home	50		82	92	
	hospital	51		63		
Nigeria	home		56	79	87	
	hospital	44	15	49	80	
Zaire	home	75		77	59	
	hospital	64		77	24	
Chile	home			14	61	
	hospital	60		53	64	
Guatemala	home			30	43	
	hospital	12		6	6	
India	home	18	19	14	14	
	hospital	10	22	15	19	
Philippines	home	40		41	31	
	hospital	18		9	8	
Hungary	hospital					41
Sweden	hospital					73

[a] See footnote to Table 1.

of interpreting the phrase "never breast-fed", it is not possible to exclude cases in which breast-feeding was not attempted, and the figures are accordingly based on all cases. However, since the proportions of "never breast-fed" infants were high only in the A groups of Guatemala and the Philippines, the inclusion of "never breast-fed" cases is likely to have little influence on the conclusions.

In countries where home deliveries were usual, it was evident that the early initiation of breast-feeding was generally more common in the case of such deliveries than in that of hospital deliveries (see Table 26). Among the urban poor in Ethiopia, for example, the difference was highly significant.

Among mothers delivered in hospital, there were large differences between countries with respect to the prevalence of early breast-feeding, the percentages ranging from 6 % to 80 %.

Table 27 Percentage of mothers breast-feeding by age of child, according to whether the child was first put to the breast within 12 hours of delivery or later*

Country	Group [a]	Time of first breast-feeding	Age of child (months)		
			0–2	3–5	6–8
			%	%	%
Ethiopia	A	<12 h	76	65	28
		later	74	33	24
	C	<12 h	100	95	90
		later	90	74	69
Chile	A	<12 h	78	43	21
		later	65	15	16
	C	<12 h	89	65	49
		later	77	66	38
	R	<12 h	92	80	57
		later	80	54	36
Guatemala	A	<12 h	47	12	6
		later	50	13	5
	C	<12 h	90	83	78
		later	82	61	63
	R	<12 h	97	100	100
		later	93	95	93
Hungary	All	<12 h	76	38	20
		later	67	31	15
Sweden	All	<12 h	80	44	23
		later	52	17	28

* Groups in which no differences were discernible are omitted.
[a] See footnote to Table 1.

In the great majority of cases, early initiation of breast-feeding was associated with a higher prevalence of subsequent breast-feeding. Table 27 summarizes the percentages of mothers breast-feeding, by age of child and according to whether the child was put to the breast within the first 12 hours or later. The differences are significant in the case of Hungary.

Mothers working during lactation

Since breast-feeding behaviour might be influenced by work demands, mothers were classified according to whether they had been in paid employment during the month preceding the interview; full-time work was differentiated from part-time work. Interviewers recorded "not applicable" in the case of mothers who were not normally paid for work (e.g., those engaged in subsistence farming) and those not working during paid maternity leave.

It should be noted that the question refers to paid work and does not cover other kinds of unpaid activity which nevertheless involve work

Table 28. Percentage of mothers working for payment, full-time (FT) or part-time (PT), by age of child*

Country	Group[a]	Age of child (months)					
		0–5		6–11		12 or more	
		FT	PT	FT	PT	FT	PT
		%	%	%	%	%	%
Ethiopia	A	82	0	87	0	92	0
	C	38	9	53	6	55	8
	R	9	26	17	37	13	32
Nigeria	A	94	0	87	0		
	B	67	0	77	0	94	0
	C	3	5	3	7	2	10
	R	0	0	0	0	1	2
Guatemala	A	25	1	32	1	37	0
	C	67	0	71	0	78	0
India	A	74	4	83	0	94	6
	B	95	4	96	0	93	0
	C	71	23	62	37	48	47
	R	100	0	99	98	2	0
Philippines	A	78	12	67	25	75	15
	C	14	22	41	22	39	29
	R	3	52	23	67	31	59
Hungary	all	0	0	6	0	7	1
Sweden	all	1	1	15	36		

* Mothers who were not normally paid for work and those on maternity leave are excluded.
[a] See footnote to Table 1.

outside the home. This may be important, for example, in Zaire, where it is usual for rural mothers to work in the fields, taking their babies with them.

As can be seen from Table 28, in Ethiopia most A-group mothers returned to full-time work soon after delivery; in the C and R groups the proportions were much lower, and in the R group part-time work predominated. In Nigeria, more than 90 % of A-group mothers returned to full-time work within 3 months of delivery; the percentages for the B group were also high. In the urban-poor (C) group, some mothers were employed in part-time work, fewer in full-time work. In the rural group, paid work appeared to be very unusual.

In Guatemala most mothers who worked did so on a full-time basis; about one-third of mothers in the A group returned to work after 3 months, the proportion showing little increase with age of child. In the C and R groups, considerably higher percentages of mothers returned to work soon after delivery, but, on the whole, the actual numbers were low.

In the Philippines, there were highly significant differences between groups. Nearly all A-group mothers returned to work (usually full-time) soon after delivery; in the other two groups, the proportions returning were also high, but part-time work was more common in the case of the rural group. In India, on the other hand, differences between groups were small; about 70 % of mothers in all groups (excluding those to whom the question was not applicable) returned to paid work post partum; in the C group part-time work was common.

In Hungary, because of legislation providing for maternity leave and job security, the percentages of mothers returning to work during the first year were low. This was also true in Sweden for the first 6 months; but, by the end of the first year, nearly 20 % of mothers in Sweden had returned to full-time work and nearly half to part-time work.

The percentages of mothers breast-feeding according to work situation are based on all working mothers (full- and part-time) and on all those not reported to be working (including "not applicable" responses). Because of the small numbers in one or other category, meaningful comparisons could be made only in the cases of Sweden and the R group in India, in which there was no difference in the prevalence of breast-feeding between working and non-working mothers. However, if age groups are amalgamated, certain trends do emerge and, as can be seen from Fig. 7, the prevalence tended to be consistently higher among non-working mothers.

Summary of findings

In general, no association was found between the prevalence of breast-feeding and the age and parity of the mother. In Sweden, maternal educational level was positively correlated with breast-feeding; in other countries, such trends as were observed tended to be in the opposite direction.

Fig. 7. Percentage of mothers breast-feeding, by employment status and age of child

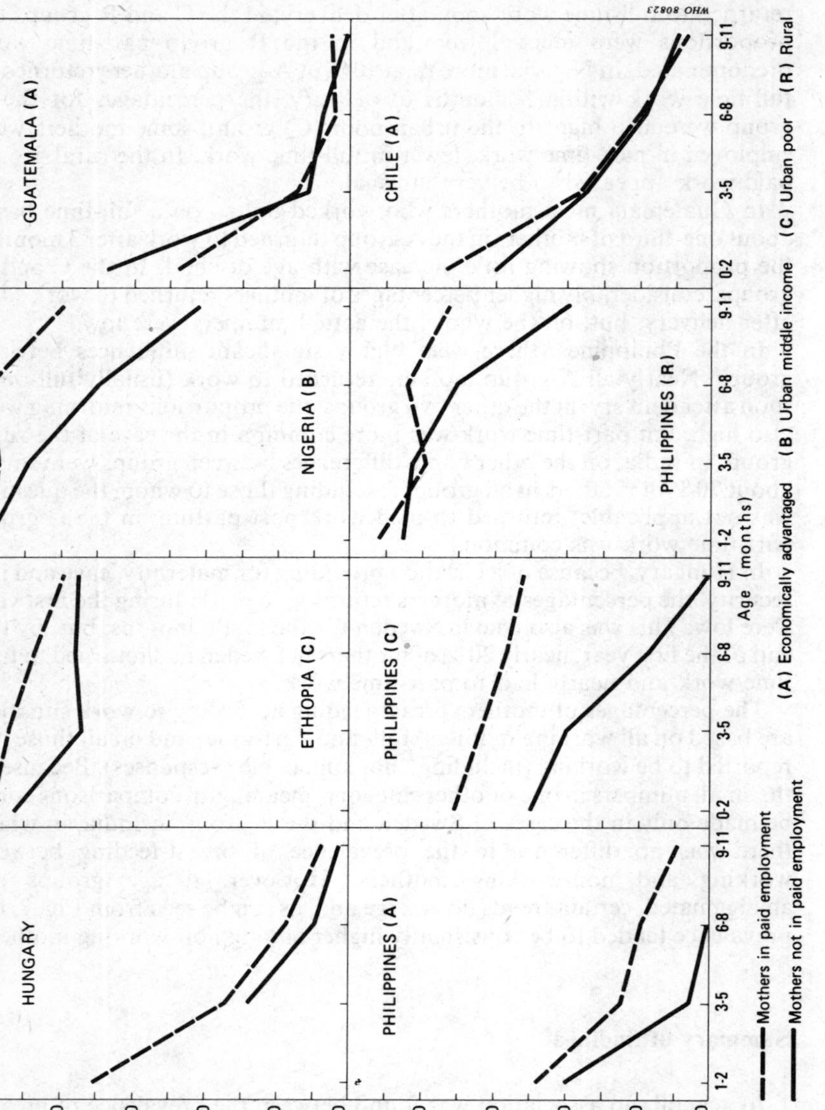

No significant associations were found between prevalence of breast-feeding and the length of time mothers had resided at their present address.

Except in Guatemala, no association was observed between the prevalence of breast-feeding and the type of family (nuclear or extended).

There was no evidence of any association between the prevalence of breast-feeding and maternal health during pregnancy as assessed by the mother herself.

It was not possible to determine the influence that place of delivery had on breast-feeding in most of the groups studied, because the patterns of delivery within groups were often too homogeneous. In Sweden and Chile, the prevalence of breast-feeding was higher among mothers whose babies had "roomed-in".

Provision of free milk samples and feeding-bottles to mothers while they were in hospital was not uncommon among some groups in Nigeria, Guatemala, and the Philippines. In Guatemala, breast-feeding was less common among those who had received such gifts; in the Philippines, too, the practice may be associated with the high proportion of economically advantaged mothers who did not breast-feed. However, among the rural group in the Philippines, there was no obvious association between the provision of free samples and breast-feeding.

The timing of the first breast-feed followed no uniform pattern. In this respect, practices varied considerably between countries and groups. The initiation of breast-feeding within the first 12 hours appeared to be associated with a higher prevalence of breast-feeding.

The data suggest that mothers who did not return to work tended to breast-feed for longer than those who did go back to gainful employment.

7. Birth weight, weight gain in infancy, and mortality among previous children

In this chapter, data are presented on the birth weights of the children in the study and their weights at the time the mothers were interviewed. These weights are, in turn, related to WHO reference values. Patterns of infant mortality in the groups studied are also considered.

Birth weight

The mean birth weights of the index children[1] are presented in Table 29. These data were provided by the mothers at the time of interview and, where possible, were checked against available birth records.

As expected, in most groups, the mean birth weights for males were higher than those for females. Taking both sexes together, the highest mean birth weight (3.5 kg) was reported in Sweden and the lowest (2.9 kg) among the urban poor in the Philippines and the rural poor in Guatemala.

Mean birth weights for economically advantaged groups were around 3.3 kg in Africa and in Chile and around 3.1 kg in Asia and in Guatemala. Means for the urban-poor groups, and for the B group in India, were consistently lower than those for the urban economically advantaged groups.

There are marked differences between countries and groups in the reported percentages of babies of low birth weight (LBW).[2] In Sweden, and among the urban economically advantaged and middle-income groups of Nigeria, about 4% of the index children weighed 2.5 kg or less at birth; in the rural group of Zaire and the economically advantaged and middle-income groups of India, on the other hand, the proportion was about 18%. Among the rural population of Guatemala it was 25%. Within most countries for which information is available, the percentage of LBW infants was consistently lower among the economically advantaged than

[1] By definition these are the children who survived. The data on low birth weight are therefore underestimates of its real incidence.

[2] Birth weight equal to or below 2500 g.

Table 29. Birth weights of index children, means and standard deviations (SD) in kg, and percentage in each group weighing 2.5 kg or less*

Country	Group[a]	Boys			Girls			Both			Percentage ≤ 2.5 kg
		mean	SD	no.	mean	SD	no.	mean	SD	no.	
		kg			kg			kg			
Ethiopia	A	3.36	0.51	141	3.24	0.58	135	3.30	0.55	276	7.9
Nigeria	A	3.37	0.48	129	3.23	0.42	104	3.31	0.45	233	4.3
	B	3.36	0.41	268	3.39	0.44	202	3.37	0.42	470	3.1
Zaire	A	3.32	0.53	287	3.22	0.54	268	3.27	0.54	555	7.0
	C	3.35	0.54	208	3.25	0.51	183	3.30	0.53	391	8.2
	R	3.09	0.51	180	3.05	0.62	166	3.07	0.56	346	17.6
Chile	A	3.37	0.46	139	3.24	0.46	156	3.30	0.47	295	5.4
	C	3.22	0.50	149	3.15	0.49	145	3.18	0.50	294	8.8
	R	3.27	0.49	216	3.09	0.55	196	3.18	0.53	412	10.9
Guatemala	A	3.19	0.45	307	3.12	0.45	284	3.15	0.45	591	6.9
	C	3.14	0.49	281	3.01	0.51	253	3.08	0.50	534	13.3
	R	2.93	0.55	131	2.94	0.52	115	2.94	0.53	246	24.8
India	A	3.12	0.53	378	3.06	0.50	382	3.09	0.51	760	16.2
	B	3.07	0.56	304	2.99	0.52	307	3.03	0.54	611	18.8
Philippines	A	3.18	0.51	257	3.03	0.49	230	3.11	0.50	487	11.9
	C	2.96	0.57	306	2.91	0.57	271	2.93	0.57	577	22.9
Hungary	all	3.27	0.52	4106	3.11	0.49	3844	3.19	0.51	7950	9.2
Sweden	all	3.55	0.54	303	3.44	0.53	292	3.50	0.54	595	3.9

* Groups with low response rates are excluded.
[a] See footnote to Table 1.

among the urban poor, and lower among the urban poor than among the rural population.

Birth weight and breast-feeding

No evidence was found of a relationship between birth weight and the prevalence of breast-feeding in Ethiopia, Nigeria, Zaire, Guatemala, or India, but among the urban population in the Philippines there was some suggestion that LBW babies were less likely to be breast-fed; the numbers involved, however, were small. In Hungary, Sweden, and Chile, differences in breast-feeding according to whether the baby was LBW or not became apparent at 3 months (see Table 30).

Table 30. Percentage of children breast-feeding at 3 months, by birthweight (retrospective data)*

Country	Group[a]	Birth weight	
		≤2.5 kg	>2.5 kg
		%	%
Chile	A	27	51
	C	59	74
	R	58	81
Hungary	all	45	55
Sweden	all	37	61

* Omitting groups in which differences were either not apparent or not significant.
[a] See footnote to Table 1.

Weight of child at time of interview

All the index children were weighed by a standardized method at the time of interview.

The data presented in Table 31, along with those in Annex 1, Table A4, giving the mean weights by age of child, have been used to construct a series of growth curves for the different groups studied in which the calculated weights are plotted against the WHO reference values (Fig. 8 a-g).[1]

In Hungary and Sweden, and in the economically advantaged groups of Ethiopia, Nigeria, Chile, and Guatemala, the average weights were

[1] WORLD HEALTH ORGANIZATION, *A growth chart for international use in maternal and child health care*, Geneva, 1978.

Table 31. Weights of index children (both sexes) by age, means and standard deviations (SD) in kg*

Country	Group[a]	Age (months)											
		1		3		6		9		12–14		18–20	
		mean	SD	mean	SD	mean	SD	mean	SD	mean	SD	mean	SD
Ethiopia	A	4.6	0.4 (8)	6.4	0.9 (20)	7.5	1.0 (15)	9.1	1.2 (13)	10.7	1.9 (22)	11.6	1.9 (25)
	C	4.1	0.9 (36)	5.4	1.0 (32)	6.7	1.1 (27)	7.6	1.0 (31)	8.5	1.4 (78)	9.3	1.6 (50)
	R			5.2	0.9 (29)	6.4	1.0 (17)	7.0	1.2 (48)	8.0	1.4 (91)	9.1	1.5 (62)
Nigeria	A	4.6	0.9 (20)	6.3	0.9 (23)	7.9	1.5 (19)	9.1	1.2 (20)				
	B	4.5	0.9 (25)	5.4	1.0 (23)	7.0	1.2 (23)	8.3	0.8 (22)	10.6	1.5 (70)	12.6	2.1 (73)
	C	3.7	1.1 (25)	5.5	1.1 (26)	6.4	1.2 (35)	7.6	1.4 (30)	8.2	1.2 (79)	9.0	1.2 (77)
	R	4.1	0.6 (26)	5.4	0.8 (27)	6.2	1.2 (27)	7.2	0.8 (29)	8.6	1.2 (90)	9.9	1.3 (78)
Chile	A	4.0	0.7 (25)	6.0	0.7 (25)	7.6	1.1 (24)	9.5	1.5 (23)				
	C	3.7	0.5 (24)	5.4	0.7 (25)	7.2	1.1 (22)	8.5	1.1 (24)				
	R	3.8	0.6 (25)	5.5	0.9 (25)	7.0	1.0 (24)	8.4	1.2 (23)	9.3	1.0 (74)		
Guatemala	A	4.3	0.6 (52)	6.1	0.7 (39)	8.1	1.0 (44)	8.9	0.9 (22)	10.6	1.5 (32)	10.7	0.9 (10)
	C	4.7	1.1 (21)	5.7	1.2 (15)	7.0	1.2 (18)	8.1	1.4 (19)	8.9	1.4 (59)	9.8	1.2 (52)
	R	4.4	0.9 (18)	5.6	0.7 (28)	6.9	0.9 (24)	7.6	0.9 (22)	8.1	1.0 (65)	8.9	1.4 (47)
India	A	4.0	0.8 (34)	5.8	1.0 (37)	7.6	0.9 (34)	8.8	1.3 (32)	9.7	1.5 (117)	10.6	1.4 (81)
	B	3.7	0.5 (34)	5.4	1.0 (38)	7.0	0.8 (42)	7.8	1.1 (43)	9.2	1.6 (123)	9.9	1.3 (82)
	C	3.9	0.7 (33)	5.1	0.9 (32)	6.1	1.0 (56)	7.1	1.2 (36)	7.5	1.2 (122)	8.3	1.3 (84)
	R	3.7	0.7 (46)	4.9	0.7 (50)	6.1	0.9 (54)	6.8	0.9 (47)	7.5	1.1 (223)	8.1	1.1 (136)
Philippines	A	4.5	1.5 (31)	6.8	1.2 (25)	7.6	1.6 (30)	8.7	1.3 (22)	9.9	1.4 (55)	10.4	1.3 (38)
	C	4.1	0.6 (36)	5.7	1.0 (46)	6.7	0.9 (45)	7.4	1.2 (29)	8.2	1.0 (94)	8.9	1.0 (89)
	R	4.1	0.7 (49)	6.1	1.0 (35)	7.2	0.9 (28)	7.9	1.1 (36)	8.3	1.1 (93)	9.2	1.2 (85)
Hungary	all	3.9	0.7 (615)	5.5	0.8 (615)	7.5	1.0 (763)	8.8	1.1 (658)				
Sweden	all	4.7	0.5 (49)	6.1	0.6 (50)	7.8	0.9 (50)	9.4	1.0 (49)				

* Figures in parentheses indicate the numbers of children in each category; the numbers for Zaire were too small to be included.

[a] See footnote to Table 1.

generally up to standard. In the Indian A group, however, the average weights at all ages were slightly below those in the A groups of other countries, and mean values after the first year were also lower in the Philippine A group. In Nigeria and India, average weights of children in the middle-income groups were appreciably lower than those of children from economically advantaged backgrounds until the age of 12 months. In Nigeria, however, they caught up with, and even exceeded, the reference values in the second year.

Average weights for age among most of the urban-poor and rural groups were relatively similar during the first 9 months; in general they tended to fall below the WHO reference values and below the average weights of A group children, but they were still above the third percentile. This was certainly the case for the C and R groups in Chile, although in Ethiopia, Nigeria, Guatemala, and the Philippines, they tended towards the standard third percentile. In India, the average weights of infants in the C and R groups fell well below the standard third percentile after the first 9–12 months of life.

It is noteworthy that in Nigeria, after the first year, the growth of children in the rural group tended to be superior to that of children in the urban-poor group. In Guatemala and Ethiopia, on the other hand, the reverse was the case.

In general, mean weights in all the urban-poor and rural groups were reasonably satisfactory up to about 6 months of age. After that age, except in Chile, where growth continued to be maintained among children in the two groups, all the curves for these groups fell below those for the economically advantaged groups.

Deaths among previous children

In order to define the extent of child loss, i.e., percentages of deaths among previous children in the groups studied, mothers were asked how many live children had been born to them and how many were still living.

In most of the groups the percentage of deaths increased with family size; the only exceptions to this were in Sweden (all groups), the A group in Ethiopia, and perhaps the A group in Zaire.

In most countries, infant-loss percentages generally increased progressively from the urban economically advantaged group to the urban-poor group and the rural group. Particularly high rates of child loss were reported in the C and R groups in Zaire, Ethiopia, Guatemala, and India, and in the C group in Nigeria among mothers with large families.

The relationship between infant-feeding practices and mortality among older siblings was not investigated.

Summary of findings

The proportion of infants of low birth weight was highest among the lower income groups. In Ethiopia, Nigeria, Zaire, Guatemala, and India, there was no evidence that the prevalence of breast-feeding was lower in the case of LBW babies, but in Hungary, Sweden, Chile, and, to a less marked degree, in the Philippines, the proportion of breast-feds tended to be lower among LBW babies than among those of normal birth weight; this was especially marked at 3 months post partum.

In Hungary and Sweden, and among the upper income groups of Ethiopia, Nigeria, Chile, and Guatemala, patterns of growth/weight were generally up to standard. For the most part, the growth of children in all the lower income groups tended to be satisfactory up to the age of 6 months and then slowed down. In the urban-poor and rural groups, average weights for age fell below those in the economically advantaged groups. This became particularly marked at 9–12 months in Ethiopia, Guatemala, the Philippines, and especially India.

Deaths among previous children appeared to be positively correlated with family size and inversely correlated with the socioeconomic background of the family. This was particularly noticeable in Nigeria, Ethiopia, Zaire, India, and Guatemala. Among urban-poor and rural families in the three African countries, Guatemala, and India, the proportion of deaths among previous children ranged between 19% and 32%.

Fig. 8(a)

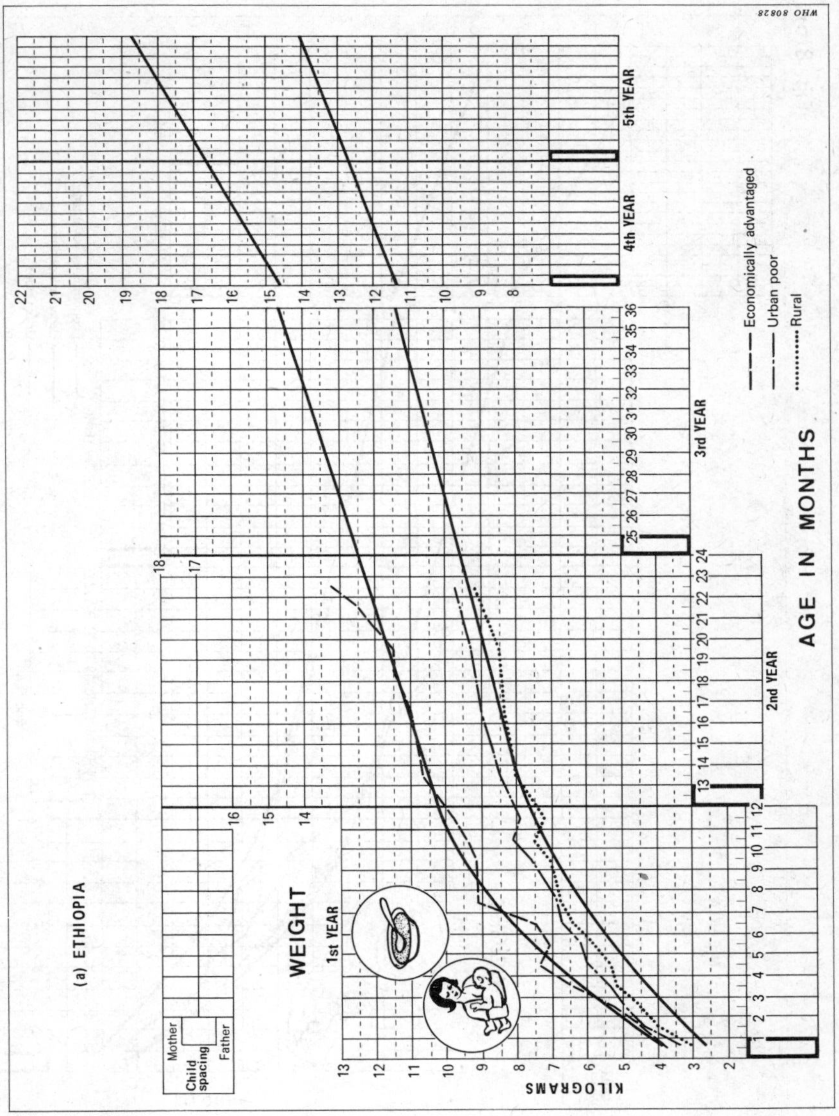

Fig. 8. Weights of index children

Fig. 8(b)

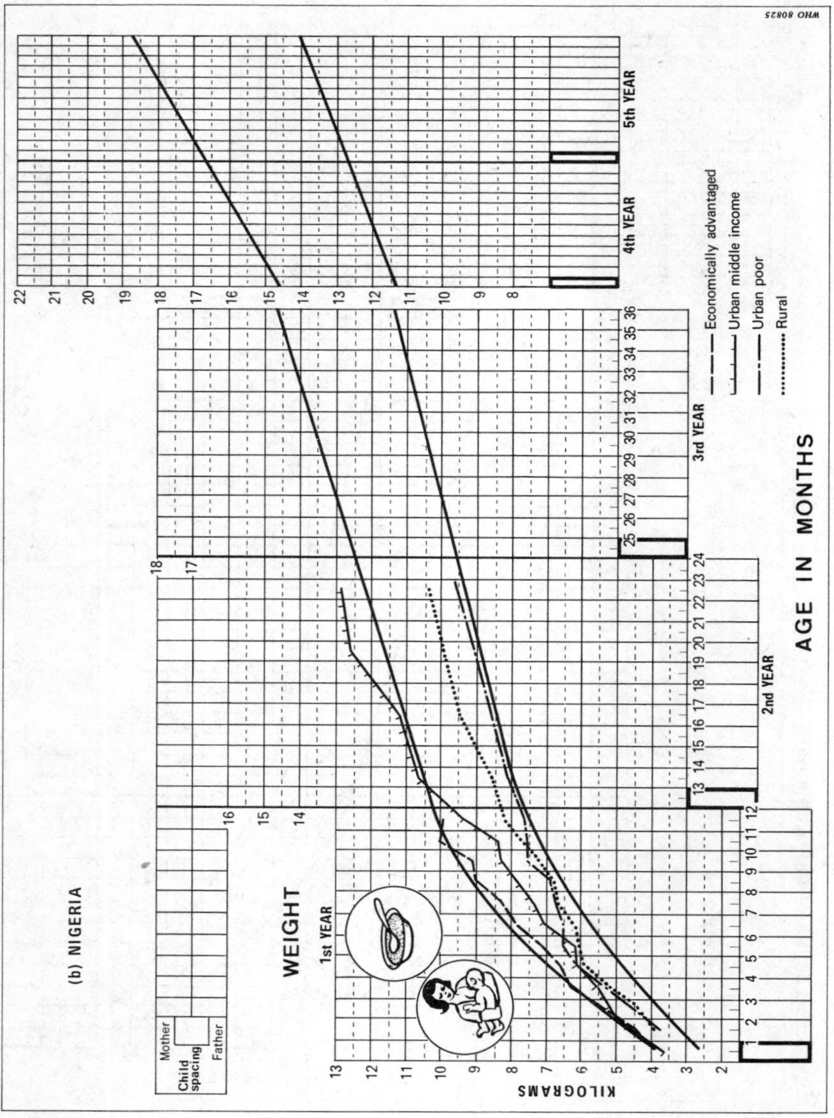
(b) NIGERIA
Child spacing
Mother
Father
WEIGHT
KILOGRAMS
1st YEAR
2nd YEAR
3rd YEAR
4th YEAR
5th YEAR
AGE IN MONTHS
Economically advantaged
Urban middle income
Urban poor
Rural
WHO 80825

Fig. 8(c)

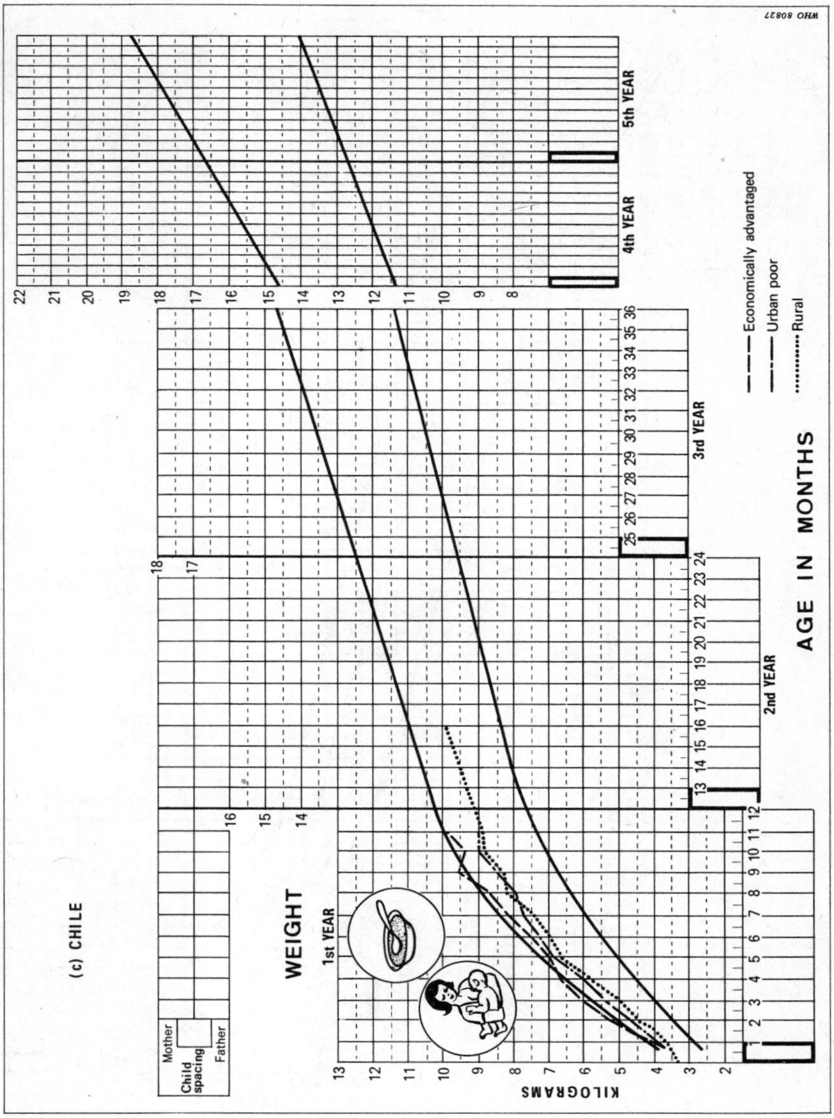
(c) CHILE
Mother
Child spacing
Father
WEIGHT
KILOGRAMS
1st YEAR
2nd YEAR
3rd YEAR
4th YEAR
5th YEAR
AGE IN MONTHS
Economically advantaged
Urban poor
Rural
WHO 80827

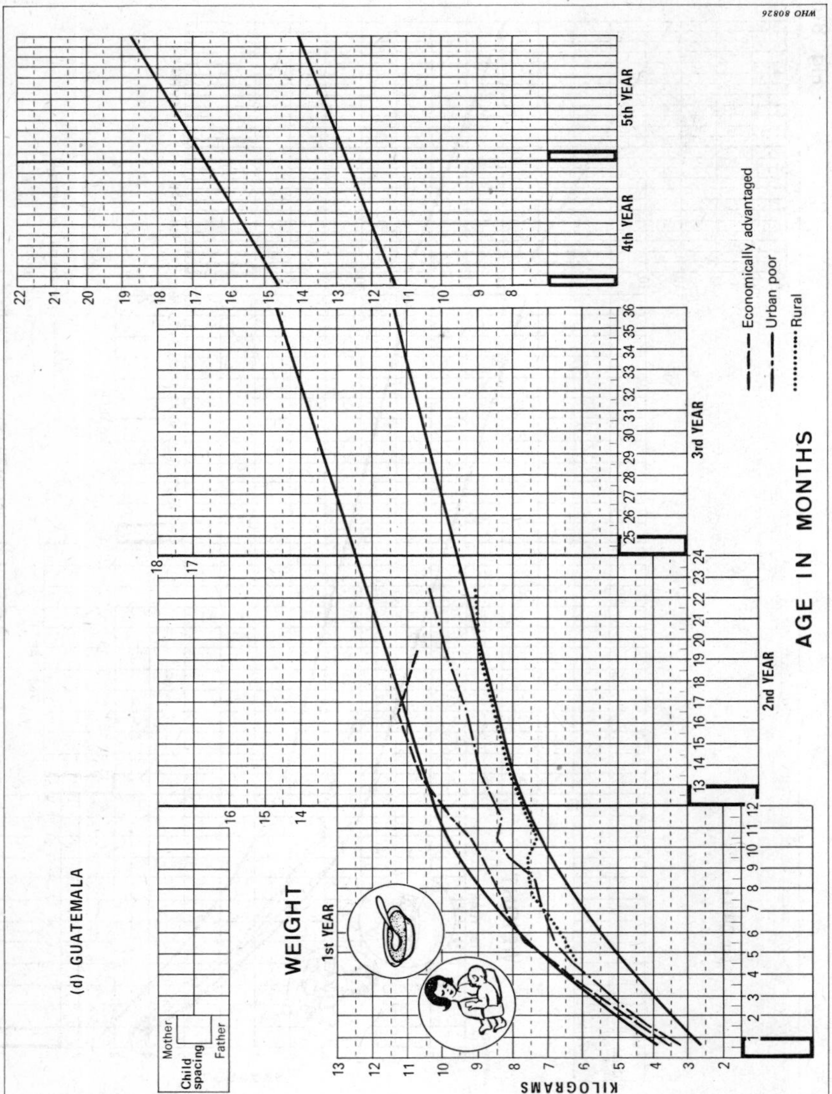
(d) GUATEMALA
Mother
Child spacing
Father
WEIGHT
1st YEAR
2nd YEAR
3rd YEAR
4th YEAR
5th YEAR
KILOGRAMS
AGE IN MONTHS
Economically advantaged
Urban poor
Rural
WHO 80826

Fig. 8(d)

Fig. 8(e)

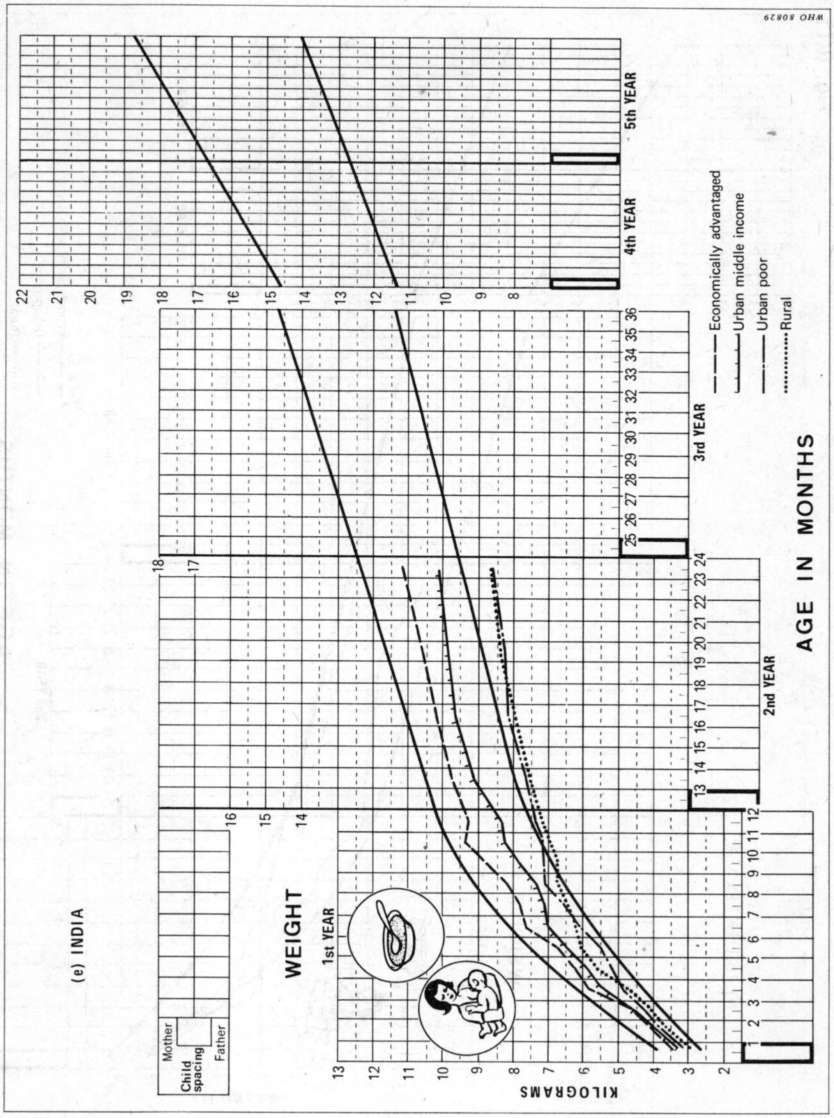
(e) INDIA
Mother
Child spacing
Father
WEIGHT
KILOGRAMS
1st YEAR
2nd YEAR
3rd YEAR
4th YEAR
5th YEAR
AGE IN MONTHS
Economically advantaged
Urban middle income
Urban poor
Rural
WHO 80829

Fig. 8(f)

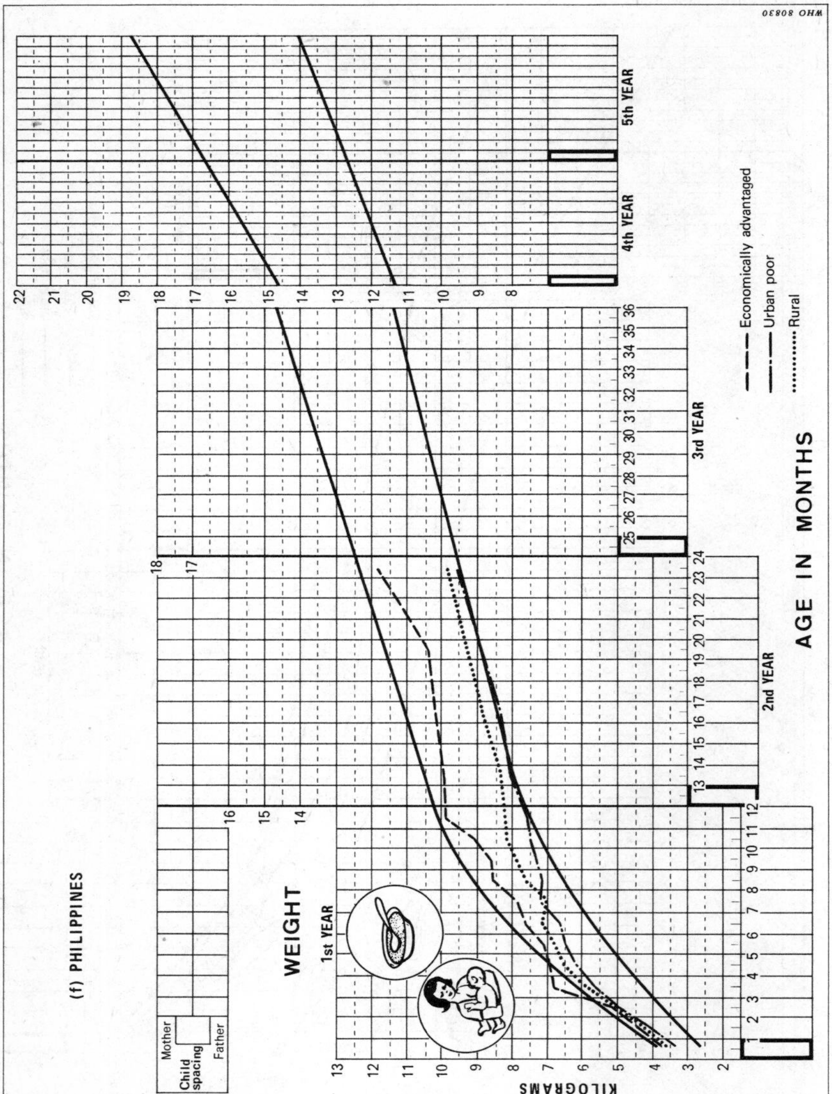

(f) PHILIPPINES
Mother
Child spacing
Father
WEIGHT
1st YEAR
2nd YEAR
3rd YEAR
4th YEAR
5th YEAR
KILOGRAMS
AGE IN MONTHS
Economically advantaged
Urban poor
Rural
WHO 80830

Fig. 8(g)

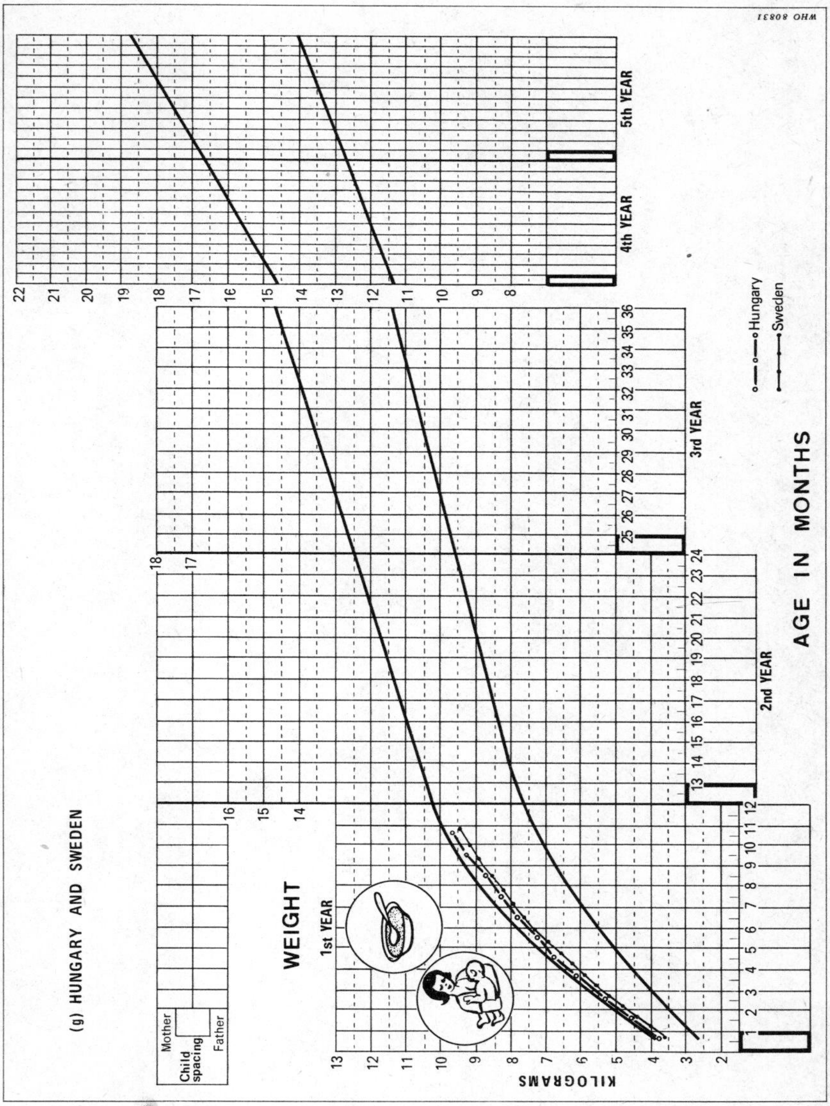
(g) HUNGARY AND SWEDEN
Mother
Child spacing
Father
WEIGHT
KILOGRAMS
1st YEAR
2nd YEAR
3rd YEAR
4th YEAR
5th YEAR
AGE IN MONTHS
Hungary
Sweden
WHO 80831

8. Introduction of supplementary foods

This chapter reviews information concerning the proportions of breast-fed children who, at different ages, were receiving breast-milk alone or breast-milk with occasional or daily supplements. It also reviews the methods used in giving milk supplements, mothers' knowledge of brand names, the keeping of baby foods in the home, the types of supplement given, mothers' reasons for deciding to introduce supplements, and the nature of the children's diets.

Supplements to breast-feeding

Mothers who were breast-feeding were asked what supplements, if any, their children had been given in addition to breast-milk during the week preceding the interview.

Fig. 9 shows the percentage of infants who were being breast-fed exclusively (or who were receiving only minor additions such as water, fruit juices, or vitamins) at 6–7 months. The data illustrated by this figure are included in Table 32.

At 6 and 7 months, 61 % of the infants in the Ethiopian urban-poor group, 78 % in the Indian urban-poor group, and 88 % in the Indian rural group were receiving no substantial additions to breast-milk. Other groups in which relatively high proportions of infants were not regularly given any supplementary foods were the Guatemalan rural group and the Indian middle-income group.

Table 33 gives the percentages of infants receiving occasional or regular supplements to breast-milk at 2–3, 6–7, and 12–13 months. The supplements given included milk, milk-based products, and various solid foods in significant amounts. In all groups except the R group in Guatemala and the C and R groups in India, one-third or more of the mothers had introduced supplementary feeding—more frequently on a regular than on an occasional basis—by the time the child was 3 months old. The prevalence of supplementation usually rose steeply with child age, and, except in the C and R groups in Ethiopia and India, nearly all mothers were giving regular supplements by 12–13 months. However, at 18 months, 20 % of mothers in the C group in India were still not giving supplements to breast-milk.

More detailed data on supplementation are given in Annex 1, Table A5.

Types of supplement given to breast-fed infants

All mothers were asked what foods their child was being given. The following categories were used in recording the answers: milk or milk-based products, cereals, animal products other than milk, legumes, vegetables, low-cost protein-rich weaning foods, "other foods".

The information derived from this question is extensive but difficult to interpret in nutritional terms in the absence of data on the quantities of

Fig. 9. Percentage of breast-fed children receiving breast-milk alone at 6 and 7 months*

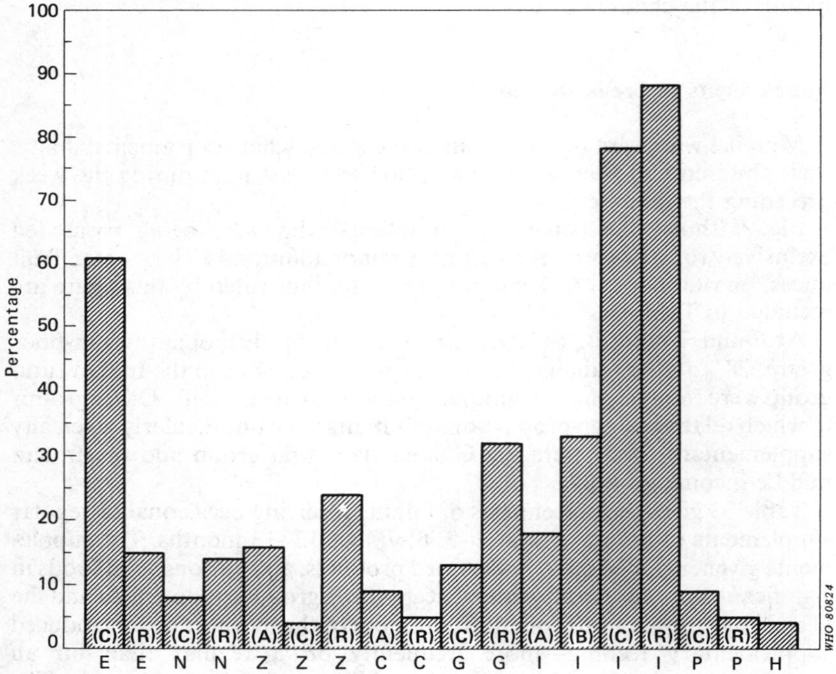

E: Ethiopia N: Nigeria Z: Zaire C: Chile
G: Guatemala I: India P: Philippines H: Hungary

(A) Economically advantaged (B) Urban middle income (C) Urban poor (R) Rural

*"Breast-milk alone" includes breast-milk with only minor additions (e.g., water, fruit juice, or vitamins).

Table 32. Percentage of breast-fed children receiving breast-milk alone, by age*

Country	Group[a]	Age of child (months)		
		6–7	12–13	18 or more
		%	%	%
Ethiopia	A			
	C	61	15	12
	R	15	6	1
Nigeria	A	0		
	B	0		
	C	8	4	2
	R	14	2	1
Zaire	A	16	0	0
	C	4	9	1
	R	24	2	0
Chile	A	9		
	C	0		
	R	5	0	
Guatemala	A			
	C	13	0	0
	R	34	0	0
India	A	18	0	0
	B	33	9	0
	C	78	40	20
	R	88	36	5
Philippines	A			
	C	9	0	0
	R	5	3	0
Hungary	all	4		
Sweden	all	0		

* "Breast-milk alone" includes breast-milk with only minor additions. (e.g., water, fruit juice or vitamins).

[a] See footnote to Table 1.

food given and the precise times when the foods were introduced into the children's diets. It does, however, indicate the general patterns in the different areas studied.

Ethiopia

Nearly all supplements given in the first year included milk or milk-based products; in the A and R groups, this form of supplementation continued after the first year of life, but in the C group it fell off sharply. Cereals were introduced during the first 3 months in the case of about one-third of the babies receiving supplements in the R group, and during the second

Table 33. Percentage of breast-feeding mothers giving occasional supplements (OS) or regular supplements (RS), by age of child

Country	Group[a]	Age of child (months) 2–3		6–7		12–13	
		OS	RS	OS	RS	OS	RS
		%	%	%	%	%	%
Ethiopia	A	11	57				
	C	16	33	16	23	39	46
	R	18	31	32	53	51	43
Nigeria	A	0	86	0	100		
	B	0	98	0	100		
	C	0	63	2	90	2	94
	R	0	35	0	86	0	98
Zaire	A	11	28	22	62	10	90
	C	4	32	13	83	17	74
	R	14	35	4	72	0	98
Chile	A	0	60	0	91		
	C	0	59	0	100		
	R	3	56	0	95	0	100
Guatemala	A	0	91				
	C	0	52	0	87	0	100
	R	2	12	4	62	0	100
India	A	3	49	3	79	4	96
	B	6	24	1	66	2	89
	C	0	6	3	19	6	54
	R	0	2	0	12	2	62
Philippines	A	39	46				
	C	13	23	9	82	0	100
	R	13	29	18	77	10	87
Hungary	all	14	33	27	69		
Sweden	all	4	27	3	97		

[a] See footnote to Table 1.

3 months to those in the A and C groups. Cereals were given by the end of the first year to nearly all babies receiving supplements in the A group, and by the end of the second year to those in the C and R groups. Animal products were given to about one-quarter of babies in all groups at 6–8 months and to nearly all babies in the A group by 9–11 months. In the C group, about 60 % received extra animal products during the second year; in the rural group, the proportion was 20 %. About half of all mothers in the A group said they gave legumes during the first 6 months, and they were given by about half the mothers in the C and R groups during the second year.

Nigeria

Between 90% and 100% of all babies who received supplementary foods were given extra milk or milk-based products during the first 3 months. In the C and R groups, the frequency of milk and milk-based supplements decreased with child age to about 50% after 6 months; in the A and B groups, however, it remained high. In the A group, 22% of the babies receiving supplements were given cereals during the first 3 months, the proportion for other groups being about 10%. In all groups, by the end of the first year, nearly all babies receiving supplements were being given cereals. Animal products were given most frequently in the A group, being introduced in about 10% of cases during the first 3 months and in more than two-thirds of all cases after 6 months; in the remaining groups, only 35–55% of the babies receiving supplements were given any animal products by 9–11 months. Legumes were introduced gradually, but by the end of the first year they were being given to about half of the babies receiving supplements. In 25% of families in all groups, vegetables were given during the second 3 months, the proportions increasing rather slowly with age in the C and R groups.

Zaire

During the first year, milk and milk-based products were given to less than half the babies receiving supplements in the A group, and the proportions declined during the second year. In the C and R groups, milk was rarely used at all. During the first 6 months, cereals were given more widely in the C and R groups than in the A group, the relevant proportions being 60%, 70%, and 45% respectively, but during the second year their use increased to 80–90% in all groups. In all groups, animal products were given, by 6–8 months, to about 30% of babies receiving supplements, the proportion rising to about 90% by 18 months. Legumes were introduced during the second 3 months into the diets of about half the babies in the A and C groups and at the end of the first year into those of 80% of the babies in the R group. Vegetables and fruits were introduced by about one-third of mothers in all groups within 3 months, and by the end of the first year their use was nearly universal.

Chile

Milk and milk-based products were given to 75–90% of babies receiving supplements in the first 3 months, their use falling during the latter part of the first year and then tending to rise in the R group (the only Chilean study group in which the study period extended beyond 1 year). Of the babies receiving supplements, 20% of those in the A group, 48% of those in the C group, and 62% of those in the R group were given cereals during the second 3 months; these proportions increased with time. Cereals, animal products, or legumes were even given to babies aged under 3 months. On the other hand, nearly all those given supplements got animal products and vegetables after 6 months and legumes after 9 months of age.

Guatemala

During the first 3 months, milk was used in the diet of more than 75% of babies receiving supplements, but the proportion declined sharply after that, particularly in the C and R groups. Cereals were introduced during the first 3 months and were being given after 6 months to nearly all babies receiving supplements. Practically no other supplementary foods were specified by name during the first 3 months; "other supplements" (nature not specified in tabulations) were, however, mentioned by 12% of mothers in the A group and 22% in the B group. Animal products were given to more than half the babies receiving supplements after 6 months. On the whole, legumes were introduced more gradually and, in fact, they were not used extensively by mothers in the R group at any age. In the A group, vegetables were introduced at an early stage, being given after the third month to nearly all babies receiving supplements. In the C and R groups, most mothers were giving their babies vegetables by 9 months. Low-cost protein foods such as Incaparina were given to 30–40% of babies receiving supplements in the C and R groups after the first 3 months, and "other supplements" were used rather extensively by all groups after the third month.

India

As already noted, the proportion of babies in the urban-poor and rural groups who were given supplements of any kind was low. Among those that were, milk and milk-based products were common in all groups during the first 6 months. The proportion of babies given milk remained high (about 90% and 75% respectively) in the A and B groups throughout the first 18 months; in the other two groups over the same period there was a sharp decrease (to about 40% in the C group and 20% in the R group). Cereals were not commonly used during the first 6 months, but were being given to about 90% of babies receiving supplements in all groups by the early part of the second year. Other foods were very rarely used during the first 6 months. Even in the A group, less than half the babies receiving supplements were given animal products other than milk, and the proportions were still lower in the B, C, and R groups. Legumes were most used after 6 months by mothers in the R group (in 80–90% of cases after 9–11 months) but the proportions were somewhat lower in the A, B, and C groups.

Vegetables were seldom used by mothers in the C group. Less than 25% of mothers in this group reported them as part of their babies' diets at any age; but, by 12 months, they were given by nearly all mothers in the A group, about three-quarters of those in the B group, and about half of those in the R group. Of the mothers giving foods other than breast-milk after 9 months, about one-third of those in the A group and smaller proportions in the remaining groups referred to "other supplements". Low-cost proteins were used by a very small minority of mothers, mainly in the C group.

Philippines

Milk and milk-based products were given to more than 90% of babies receiving supplements in all groups during the first 3 months, their use decreasing to about 50% in the second year. During the first 3 months, cereals were given to about one-third of babies receiving supplements in group A, but to very few in the other groups. By 6 months, however, nearly all the babies receiving supplements were being given cereals of one kind or another. No other supplementary foods were given to breast-fed babies in the first 3 months, except in the A group, in which 20% of babies receiving supplements were given animal products or vegetable supplements; by 9 months, however, about 80% were receiving animal products or vegetables and about 35% were receiving legumes. Low-cost protein supplements were also given to about 20% of group-C babies receiving supplements, after they reached 6 months of age.

Hungary

About 90% of the babies who were being given supplementary foods were given milk or milk-based products within 2 months of birth. This proportion decreased with age as other supplements were introduced, but about three-quarters were still receiving some milk or milk-based supplements at the end of the first year. Cereals were usually introduced during the second 3 months of life and were being given to about 75% of babies at 1 year. Animal products (other than milk) and, to a lesser extent, legumes were being given to about 75% by 1 year. Vegetables were given to some 20% within the first 3 months and to nearly all older babies.

Sweden

All babies whose diets involved some supplementation received milk-based products within 3 months of birth and very occasionally, vegetable preparations. No other supplements were used at this stage. Animal protein and legumes were given to 30–40% of babies in their second 3 months of life and to nearly all babies by 9 months. Vegetables were usually given from 3 months onwards and cereals from 6 months onwards.

Methods of feeding with milk or milk-based formulas

Mothers were asked to specify how they fed their infants with milk and milk-based products; their responses evidently depended on the age of the child at the time of the interview. However, in nearly all countries and groups, mothers used bottles, at least initially; only in the R groups in Ethiopia and India (77% and 40% respectively) was there a tendency towards "hand-feeding". The use of spoons and cups increased at later ages.

Child weight and supplementation

The survey produced no evidence of consistent differences in weight-for-age between breast-fed and non-breast-fed babies; similarly, within the breast-fed group, there was no difference between those receiving or not receiving supplements. While, in Hungary, breast-fed babies receiving supplements were consistently heavier from 6 months onwards than similar babies not receiving them, an examination of the weight gains from birth shows no differences to account for this, and the finding must be regarded with some caution.

It is worth noting, however, that among groups (such as the C and R groups in India) in which supplements were introduced at a rather late stage (after 6 months), there was also evidence of unusually flat growth curves. Although it is not possible to demonstrate that these two phenomena are causally related, it is extremely likely that they are.

Reasons for regular supplementation

The question on mothers' reasons for introducing regular supplementation when they did was "open-ended", and they were allowed to give more than one reason. The types of responses varied considerably, and they are difficult to classify. Consequently, only the main "types" of response are outlined here, country by country, taking into account the age of the child at the time when regular supplementation was started.

Ethiopia

There were too few responses for any analysis on this point to be undertaken.

Nigeria

Sixty-two per cent of mothers in the C group, at 0–2 months post partum, said "No particular reason"; this rose to 89% at 9 months or more. The reason for this response is not clear, since a similar reply was rarely given in any of the other study groups. "The child will grow better" was given as a reason in 47–81% of all responses from the A, B, and R groups, with no obvious change by age.

Zaire

In all groups, the two main reasons given for introducing supplements to breast-feeding were "lack of milk" and the fact that the child was crying or seemed hungry. In the A group, "lack of milk" was cited in 50% of the responses at 0–2 months post partum, the proportion falling to 35% at 6–8 months, while "child crying" or "child hungry" rose from 27% to 44% over the same period.

Chile

That the child "was hungry" accounted for about 50 % of all the responses given; there was no obvious trend by age. In the C and R groups, the proportions of mothers saying that they had started supplementation because "milk stopped" were 12 % and 22 % respectively, again without any consistent trends by age.

Guatemala

Answers such as "to improve growth", "to feed better", "to get the child used to it", "child old enough" and "child wanted other foods" accounted for about 80 % of all responses at all child ages. In addition, during the first 3 months post partum, 10–17 % of mothers said their milk was insufficient, the proportions becoming somewhat lower at later child ages.

India

Reasons such as "solids indicated", "to make baby used to solids", and "custom" accounted in the urban economically advantaged group for 11 % of all responses at 0–2 months, and for nearly 50 % of them after 6 months; the comparable changes in percentages in the B, C, and R groups are 6–35 %, 5–18 %, and 0–12 % respectively. "Insufficient milk" accounted for about 50 % of responses in the A and B groups, these percentages decreasing slightly with child age; in the C group the proportions were around 60 % throughout the age range studied; and in the R group they decreased from 83 % at 0–2 months to about half that value after 6 months.

Philippines

Reasons such as "child likes solids", "mother thinks it is important", "to train baby", and "experience" accounted for 45 %, 26 %, and 7 % of the reasons given by mothers with babies under 3 months of age in the A, C, and R groups respectively. Insufficient milk accounted for 12 %, 38 %, and 58 % respectively of responses in the three groups at 0–3 months post partum, and for 7 %–10 % at later stages.

Hungary

In all, 87 % of mothers who started supplementation during the first 3 months gave insufficient production of breast-milk as the reason; the same response was given by 41 % of mothers who began supplementation at 6–8 months.

Sweden

Insufficient milk production was given as a reason by 15 % of mothers who introduced supplements at 0–2 months post partum; at 3–5 months 9 % of mothers gave this reason, and none gave it at 6–8 months. This reason may also cover the circumstances grouped under "child hungry", "poor sucking", etc., which accounted for a further 21 % of the reasons given for supplementation at 0–2 months.

Who influenced the mothers in their decision to introduce supplementary feeds?

Mothers were asked who or what event they thought had helped them decide to begin supplementation. The answers are shown in Table 34. For the most part, medical advice appears to have been an important factor; it was quoted by between 60 % and 80 % of mothers in Hungary, Chile, and the A groups in Guatemala and the Philippines. In the A groups in Nigeria and Zaire, on the other hand, medical advice was rarely mentioned. In most of the other groups the decision to give supplements was most frequently the mother's own. Advice from husbands, friends, or from the media was not often cited in any country or group, but relatives appear to have had some influence among all study groups in the Philippines, in the C and R groups in Guatemala, and in the R group in India.

Mothers' knowledge of brand names of infant formulas

In order to obtain some indication of the spread of information on the subject, mothers were asked whether they knew the names of any commercial milk-based formulas.

In Hungary, Sweden, and all the economically advantaged and middle-income groups, most mothers knew of formula products by their brand names; this was also true of the urban-poor and rural groups in Chile, Guatemala, and the Philippines. Among the urban-poor group of Ethiopia and the rural groups of Nigeria and Zaire such knowledge was rarer and in the rural group of Ethiopia and the urban-poor and rural groups of India it was very unusual indeed.

In general, the brand names of such products were better known to mothers who were not breast-feeding than to those who were; the differences, however, were smaller than might have been expected.

Within specific groups, the mother's educational level appears to have made little difference in this respect; in fact, only in the rural group in Chile, and to some extent in the rural group in India, did education seem to be associated with knowledge of the brand names in question.

Commercial baby foods in the home

Mothers were also asked whether they had any commercial baby foods in their homes. In Table 35, the responses are shown separately for mothers who were not breast-feeding at the time of the interview, and for those who were, with and without supplementation.

Table 34. Percentage distribution of persons or influences named by mother as contributing to her decision to give supplementary foods

Country	Group[a]	Medical adviser	Relatives	Friends	Media	Other	Mother herself	Mother with father
		%	%	%	%	%	%	%
Nigeria	A	8	0	4	0	0	85	3
	B	17	3	2	0	0	72	7
	C	14	1	5	0	0	78	3
	R	13	0	6	0	0	81	1
Zaire	A	7	2	2	0	0	82	6
	C	1	2	1	0	1	89	6
	R	2	3	1	0	1	93	1
Chile	A	86	0	0	0	1	13	0
	C	67	0	0	0	3	30	0
	R	74	0	0	0	2	24	0
Guatemala	A	86	3	1	1	0	8	1
	C	53	18	5	1	4	18	1
	R	22	15	4	0	4	53	2
India	A	40	7	0	1	0	49	3
	B	31	9	0	1	0	58	1
	C	9	8	0	0	0	83	1
	R	1	21	1	0	0	75	3
Philippines	A	60	16	2	4	1	17	0
	C	18	37	5	1	2	37	0
	R	18	24	4	1	2	51	0
Hungary	all	87	1	0	0	0	12	0
Sweden	all	37	1	0	3	0	54	4

[a] See footnote to Table 1.

Table 35. Percentage of mothers with stocks of commercial baby foods in the home

Country	Group[a]	Not breast-feeding	Breast-feeding: supplemented	Breast-feeding: not supplemented
		%	%	%
Ethiopia	A	77	82	33
	C	24	17	2
	R	0	1	0
Nigeria	A	95	100	71
	B	66	92	18
	C	7	30	4
	R	2	33	1
Zaire	A	38	36	22
	C	20	12	8
	R	9	6	11
Chile	A	94	84	52
	C	63	18	23
	R	43	33	5
Guatemala	A	83	42	0
	C	9	5	0
	R	6	4	2
India	A	61	64	17
	B	42	44	5
	C	15	6	0
	R	5	0	0
Philippines	A	61	36	13
	C	18	16	4
	R	16	16	5
Hungary	all	35	38	12
Sweden	all	100	86	62

[a] See footnote to Table 1.

In most of the groups there was little difference between mothers who were not breast-feeding and those who were breast-feeding with regular supplementation. While it was to be expected that a mother feeding her child on breast-milk alone would be less likely than others to have commercial infant foods in her home, in fact there were stocks of them in the homes of more than 50% of such mothers in the A groups of Chile and Nigeria and in Sweden in general.

Summary of findings

In general, regular supplementation was started well before 6 months post partum, particularly in the economically advantaged groups. Notable exceptions were the urban-poor population groups in India and Ethiopia. in which 20% and 12% of mothers, respectively, were still breast-feeding exclusively at 18 months post partum. The types of supplementation given varied considerably, presumably depending on tradition and availability of food. For the most part milk or milk-based products were used as supplementary foods during the first 3 months. The exception was Zaire, where milk-based products were used to only a limited extent by all groups at all ages.

Where supplementary feeding was undertaken it was almost always given initially by bottle; the only exceptions were in the R groups in Ethiopia and India in which a large percentage of mothers used "hand-feeding".

Knowledge of infant foods by their brand names was extensive. Only among some urban-poor and rural groups, particularly in Ethiopia, India, Nigeria, and Zaire, did such knowledge appear to be limited.

The main reason given for introducing regular supplementation to breast-fed infants was "insufficient milk" or "hungry child". In general, the reasons given related to the mother's perception of the child's needs or her notions about when the child was ready for solids and other supplementary food.

To a large extent, it was the mothers who decided to introduce supplementary foods. In some countries, such as Hungary, Chile and Guatemala, medical advice was an important factor in their decisions.

There was no indication that the weights-for-age of breast-fed babies differed from those of non-breast-fed babies, or that supplementation was associated with weight differences. In the case of India, however, unusually flat growth curves were frequent in population groups in which it was common to delay the introduction of supplements well beyond 6 months post partum.

9. Organization of health services; social and health legislation

This chapter deals with additional survey information from the nine countries on prenatal, maternity, and postnatal services, training of health workers, legislation, and the provision of maternity leave, day care, and breaks for breast-feeding.

The information is of a general nature and refers to the areas studied; it may thus not reflect the full range of local variations or practices in other parts of the countries concerned.

Prenatal services

Prenatal care services often give mothers their first contact with formal health care or with health personnel. The setting of such services and the type of information they provide on breast-feeding have an important influence on these mothers.

As can be seen from Table 36, the range of personnel providing prenatal services varied considerably in the nine countries and, except in Hungary and Sweden, appeared to be related to the geographical location of the services.

In urban areas, and especially in the case of services used by economically advantaged groups, specialized personnel such as obstetricians were usually an integral part of the health team, together with general practitioners, nurses, and midwives.

In most rural areas, specialized personnel were relatively uncommon; in rural India and Ethiopia, pregnant women were likely to be attended by traditional midwives rather than by any other category of personnel.

There was little uniformity with respect to the number of clinic visits mothers were expected to make during pregnancy; and the figures presented in Table 36 may in some cases represent an ideal rather than the actual number of visits made by the majority of mothers. This is especially so in rural and urban-poor communities.

The type of information routinely provided as part of prenatal services often appeared to be related both to the type of health care facility and to the socioeconomic group served. There was generally less emphasis on

Table 36. Prenatal services

Country	Group[a]	Location	Personnel	Education regarding maternal/infant care	Food supplements received through health services	Frequency of service utilization
Ethiopia	A	hospital private clinic	obstetrician midwife nurse laboratory technician	Some nutrition education		Up to 7 months, monthly visits; 7–8 months, every 1–2 weeks; 8–9 months, weekly
	C	municipal clinic urban clinic	health officer midwife nurse health assistant	Demonstration sessions in municipal clinics on preparation of supplementary and home weaning foods	Soya wheat provided by municipal clinics to very poor mothers	as above
	R	health centre health clinic	midwife nurse traditional midwife community nurse	Nutrition/health education; some information on breast care		When necessary
Nigeria	A	teaching hospital hospital clinic	obstetrician physician midwife	Very little preparation for breast-feeding or nutritional counselling		Personal choice
	C	maternal and child health centre health centre	midwife nurse	Maternal/infant nutrition, breast-feeding, breast care, food preparation demonstration; sometimes commercial representatives' "milk nurses" give talks with demonstrations on infant feeding		After 4–5 months, once a month
	R	as above	as above			as above

Zaire	all	hospital health centre	nurse auxiliary nurse	General nutrition; demonstrations of child care; hygiene		Three visits before delivery by 60% of women
Chile	A	private clinic	obstetrician midwife	According to need		Up to 33 weeks, monthly visits; 33–37 weeks, every 2 weeks; remaining time, weekly
	C	outpatient clinic with referral to hospital	obstetrician midwife nurse/midwife auxiliary nurse district health team	Maternal nutrition, breast-feeding, better utilization of income on food, nutrition for lactating women, preparation of powdered milk, care of breasts	Powdered milk to all pregnant women	as above
	R	as above	as above	as above	as above	as above
Guatemala	A	private clinics	obstetrician	Some nutrition education; importance of breast-feeding		8–10 visits
	C	main health centre state hospital	resident in obstetrics physician nurse auxiliary	Care of breasts, hygiene, maternal and infant nutrition		Ideally 6–10 visits, usually 3–4 visits
	R	health centre	general nurse auxiliary traditional midwife	as above		2–14 times during pregnancy, 4–5 times in last trimester
India	A	private clinic hospital	obstetrician medical officer nurse		Vitamin and mineral tablets	Up to 28 weeks, once a month; 28–30 weeks, every 1–2 weeks; then weekly

Table 36 (*contd*)

Country	Group[a]	Location	Personnel	Education regarding maternal/infant care	Food supplements received through health services	Frequency of service utilization
India (*contd*)	C	health centre outpatient antenatal clinic	obstetrician physician nurse public health nurse auxiliary health visitor traditional midwife	Hygiene, preparation of baby kits, diet, care of breasts, breast-feeding, immunization	as above	as above
	R	primary health care centre	medical officer nurse public health nurse auxiliary health visitor traditional midwife	Preparation for home delivery, hygiene, diet, care of breasts, breast-feeding, immunization	Locally available foods (mainly solids) and foods imported by international organizations supplied to malnourished expectant mothers	as above
Philippines	A	hospital clinic	obstetrician midwife nurse assistant (recent graduate)	Information on mother's diet; breast-feeding information seldom given as it is taken for granted that these mothers will not breast-feed		1–6 months, once a month; 7–8 months, every 1–2 weeks; 9 months, weekly
	C	hospital health centre domiciliary obstetrical service team	physician midwife public health midwife student midwife nurse	Diet during pregnancy, breast-feeding advantages and patterns; care of breasts; diet for lactating mothers; child care; classes include demonstrations from commercial firms on infant feeding	Samples of vitamins, starter doses only, given to all mothers	as above

	R	rural health centre	physician public health midwife	Annual mothers' class (in accessible areas) deals with prenatal care, nutrition, breast-feeding, care of newborn, supplementary feeding, family planning		Expected to visit 3 times; most mothers attend only once before delivery
Hungary	urban	advisory dispensary	obstetrician health visitor	Nutrition during pregnancy, care of breasts, breast-feeding, infant nutrition		No fixed pattern
	rural	as above	district physician physician health visitor	as above		as above
Sweden	all	hospital maternity care centre	obstetrician midwife nurse	Maternal education group sessions on pregnancy and delivery; breast care and breast-feeding; booklets on maternal/child care provided	Iron preparations and vitamins	Up to 20 weeks, once a month; 20 weeks to 8 months, every 1–2 weeks; remaining time, weekly

[a] See footnote to Table 1.

encouraging, or preparing for, breast-feeding among economically advantaged mothers in urban areas, where advice on this point appeared to be left to the discretion of the physician and the perceived or expressed needs of the mother.

Prenatal services in urban-poor and rural communities usually included the provision of information on maternal nutrition during pregnancy, preparation for breast-feeding, care of the breasts and, in the case of Chile, information on how to optimize family expenditure for better nutrition.

In Nigeria and the Philippines, representatives of commercial infant-food companies often took part in providing educational information on infant feeding in health facilities. In Ethiopia and Sweden, it was not uncommon for educational publications for use in health facilities to be supplied by commercial food companies.

In Nigeria, sales personnel gave monthly talks to the nursing staff of maternal and child health and maternity clinics and provided information on their products. In Guatemala, salesmen often provided samples for maternity wards, and in the Philippines it was reported that salesmen were sometimes given the home addresses of new mothers.

In the Philippines and Nigeria, it was not unusual for mothers to receive "educational" visits from so-called "milk nurses" and in some cases to be given samples of products.

Maternity services

As can be seen from Table 37, in Chile, Sweden, and Hungary, hospital delivery was standard; among economically advantaged groups in the other countries it was also usual. Domiciliary delivery was common among the urban-poor and rural groups in Ethiopia, Nigeria, Zaire, and India, where traditional midwives were a major source of health care.

There was little uniformity between countries or groups concerning where the newborn infant was roomed. Much seemed to depend upon the type of health facility, its own particular policy, and whether its physical characteristics did or did not lend themselves to "rooming-in".

In Hungary all babies were routinely kept in nurseries and brought to mothers at regular intervals for feeding. This was also the case in private clinics and teaching hospitals in Nigeria. In Sweden, and in private clinics in Chile and Guatemala, the policy was to room the infant with the mother during the daytime and to separate them only during the night. In Guatemala and Chile, the tendency in hospitals and health centres providing services to the urban-poor and rural populations was to room infants with the mothers both day and night.

While, in the rural area of Zaire, it was common for infants to be roomed separately from mothers, in the urban area the reverse was true. This rural/urban difference may be partly explained by the fact that many rural health services in Zaire are operated by foreign health teams and often patterned after those of Europe and North America.

Table 37. Maternity practices

Country	Group[a]	Location	Personnel	Where infant is kept	Average duration of stay in maternity ward
Ethiopia	A	hospital private clinic	obstetrician paediatrician midwife nurse	Usually together with mother day and night	1–2 days
	C	municipal clinic	health officer midwife nurse health assistant	Together with mother day and night	6–24 hours
	R	health centre health clinic	health officer community nurse health assistant		
Nigeria	A	hospital private clinic	obstetrician paediatrician physician midwife nurse auxiliary nurse	In teaching hospitals, in nurseries	2–3 days
	C	maternity centre maternal and child health centre	as above	In maternal and child health centre, together with mother day and night	
Zaire	A	hospital clinic	physician nurse auxiliary	Hospital: generally in mother's bed; clinic: in cot in mother's room	Hospital: 4 days Clinic: 3 days

Table 37 (*contd*)

Country	Group[a]	Location	Personnel	Where infant is kept	Average duration of stay in maternity ward
Zaire (*contd*)	R	as above	auxiliary nurse	Hospital: mother and infant separated immediately; clinic: infant separated from mother for first 24 h; other practices: mother and child in same room except during morning	5–6 days
Chile	A	private clinic	obstetrician paediatrician midwife nurse auxiliary nurse	Together with mother during the day; at night in nursery	Normal delivery: 8 days
	C	hospital	as above	Usually together with mother following first breast-feed	Multipara, normal delivery: 3–4 days Primipara: 3 days Caesarian: 5 days
	R	maternity centre	as above	as above	as above
Guatemala	A	private hospital	obstetrician	In nursery	4 days
	C	public hospital social security obstetric hospital	midwife	Together with mother during the day; at night in nursery	Normal delivery: 24–36 hours Forceps: 2 days Caesarian: 5–6 days

	R	most deliveries domiciliary	traditional midwife	At home with mother	
		health centre	midwife in health centre	In same room at foot of bed in health centre	multipara: 24–30 hours primipara: 2 days
India	A	hospital private nursing home	obstetrician paediatrician neonatologist midwife nurse auxiliary nurse	Together with mother day and night	Hospital: 3 days Private nursing home: 5–7 days
	C	hospital	obstetrician paediatrician midwife nurse auxiliary nurse/midwife	as above	as above
	R	primary health care centre	medical officer auxiliary nurse/midwife traditional midwife	as above	
Philippines	A	hospital clinic	obstetrician paediatrician midwife nurse auxiliary nurse	In nursery	Normal delivery: 3–4 days Caesarian: 7 days
	C	hospital	as above	In nursery, never taken to mother	Hospital: 1–2 days
		health centre with lying-in maternity clinic	as above	In nursery	Clinic: 3 days
		domicile		Together with mother day and night	

Table 37 (*contd*)

Country	Group[a]	Location	Personnel	Where infant is kept	Average duration of stay in maternity ward
Philippines (*contd*)	R	new hospital (1976) providing services similar to those for urban elite	physician midwife nurse	In nursery	Normal delivery: 2–3 days Caesarian: 7 days
		rural health centre domiciliary service	physician (occasionally) midwife	Together with mother day and night	
		domicile	physician (occasionally) health centre midwife traditional midwife	as above	
Hungary	all	hospital maternity home	obstetrician paediatrician midwife nurse	In nursery	Hospital: 5–6 days Maternity home: 7–8 days
Sweden	all	hospital	obstetrician paediatrician midwife nurse assistant nurse nursery nurse assistant ward staff	Usually together with mother only during the day	Primipara: 6–7 days Others: 5 days Caesarian: 8–10 days

[a] See footnote to Table 1.

In urban-poor communities in the Philippines and Guatemala, and among the urban elite in Ethiopia, the average stay in hospital was 1–2 days. In Chile, India, Nigeria, the rest of the Philippines, and the urban population of Zaire, it was 2–4 days. In Hungary, Sweden, and rural Zaire, mothers tended to stay 5–7 days.

Table 38 summarizes feeding practices in hospital services in the study areas, and again shows that there was little uniformity either between countries or in different areas within countries. In Chile, for example, breast-feeding might be initiated during the first 6, 12, or 24 hours, according to the clinic or hospital. In private clinics in Guatemala, the general practice was to initiate breast-feeding at between 12 and 24 hours post partum; in the large urban hospital, breast-feeding was usually started 6 hours post partum.

In Zaire, the timing of the first breast-feed varied according to the location of the hospital; in urban areas, it was common policy for infants to be put to the breast immediately, while in rural hospitals and health centres breast-feeding was only initiated 8–24 hours after delivery. In the Philippines, breast-feeding was left to the discretion of the mother in private clinics, but in the general hospitals it was often positively discouraged. In Sweden, there is an increasing tendency to encourage the mother to initiate breast-feeding as soon after the birth as possible.

In the case of domiciliary deliveries, it was common practice to start breast-feeding almost immediately in Guatemala and Zaire, and within the first 3 hours in Nigeria and Chile. On the other hand, it might be delayed as long as 12 hours in Ethiopia and India, and up to 24 hours in the Philippines.

On-demand feeding was generally encouraged among all groups in Ethiopia, India, and Nigeria, and among the urban-poor and rural populations of Guatemala and Zaire. In Sweden, there also appeared to be a trend towards on-demand feeding, although the extent to which it was encouraged varied according to the hospital.

In Hungary and the Philippines, and in private clinics in Chile, scheduled feeding was the norm. In the Philippines, formula feeding was often recommended.

Postnatal services

Information relating to postnatal services is summarized in Table 39.

Infants in need of special care

Of special concern as far as postnatal services are concerned is the attention given to the feeding of low-birth-weight (LBW) and premature infants; information on this is presented in Table 40.

Table 38. Infant feeding practices in maternity services

Country	Group[a]	Personnel	Information given to mothers in maternity services	Initiation of breast-feeding	Feeding routines	Attitude of health personnel to breast-feeding	Activities of commercial companies	Donation distributions by commercial companies
Ethiopia	A	obstetrician nurse	Breast-care, breast-feeding techniques; in the case of working mothers bottle-feeding techniques; hygiene, child spacing	4–6 h after delivery	Breast-feeding on demand except for infants kept in the nursery	Breast-feeding encouraged	Salesmen not allowed on wards, but sometimes leave samples with head nurse	
	C	health educator nurse	Breast care, breast-feeding techniques, importance of breast-feeding, child spacing	as above	Breast-feeding on demand	as above	as above	Donations accepted for distribution to working mothers, to mothers unable to breast-feed, and to infants whose mothers have died
	R	health officer community nurse health assistant						Little if any food donated
Nigeria	A	obstetrician paediatrician physician	Breast-feeding taken for granted; information given only in response to questions	2–3 h after delivery, or when mother has recovered	On demand	Breast-feeding usually taken for granted; physician may encourage artificial feeding	In maternal and child health and maternity clinics, "milk nurses" give monthly talks on infant feeding	

	C	midwife health sister	as above	as above	as above	Breast-feeding taken for granted	as above	
Zaire	urban	obstetrician nurse	Little information given in ward; some advice when going home	Immediately after delivery unless otherwise advised	Every 4 h	Breast-feeding taken for granted		
	rural			8–24 h after delivery	On demand	as above		
Chile	A	obstetrician midwife nurse	Encouragement of breast-feeding	12 h after normal delivery, 24 h after Caesarian and forceps	Usually fixed schedule	Breast-feeding officially encouraged, but staff's attitude often indifferent	Salesmen or sales propaganda not allowed on wards	No donations accepted
	C and R	physician midwife nurse	Importance of colostrum, breast care, breast-feeding techniques, child spacing	In some hospitals, 12–18 h after normal delivery, 24 h after Caesarian or forceps; others, 6 h after normal delivery, 10 h after forceps, and 24 h after Caesarian	Varies between hospitals: only breast feeding in some, others supplement with glucose and water; infants with health problems are given powdered milk; some practise fixed schedule, others feeding on demand	Breast-feeding taken for granted	as above	Services catering for urban poor and rural population are provided with powdered milk
Guate-mala	A	physician	Encouragement of breast-feeding, but no specific policy	12–24 h after delivery in private clinics	Fixed schedule	Often indifferent to breast-feeding	Salesmen not allowed on wards but often leave samples with head nurse	

Table 38 (*contd*)

Country	Group[a]	Personnel	Information given to mothers in maternity services	Initiation of breast-feeding	Feeding routines	Attitude of health personnel to breast-feeding	Activities of commercial companies	Donation distributions by commercial companies
Guatemala (*contd*)	C	hospital staff	as above	Usually 6 h after delivery, but bottle-feeding also often introduced	On demand usually but practice varies between hospitals	Indifferent, but a more positive attitude is developing	as above	
	R	midwife auxiliary health worker	as above	Immediately	Breast-feeding on demand	Breast-feeding taken for granted		
India	A	medical officer maternity ward staff	Importance of colostrum, breast-feeding, hygiene; advised to feed every 2 h	Primiparae, 6–12 h after delivery; Others, mother's choice	On demand: glucose or sugar water usually by spoon until lactation is established; child put to breast throughout this period for colostrum	Breast-feeding greatly encouraged	No visit of salesmen	Maternity services do not accept donations, but paediatricians sometimes do
	C	as above	as above	as above	as above	as above	as above	as above
Philippines	A	obstetrician midwife nurse	Preparation of powdered milk and bottle-feeding and breast-feeding techniques, hygiene; child spacing seldom discussed	After 24 h, if mother wishes to breast-feed	Powdered milk every 3–4 h	No specific policy, staff often indifferent	Salesmen not allowed on wards, but sometimes acquire home addresses of Primiparae	Samples left with head nurse; mother takes a can of milk home

	C	public health midwife student midwife	Breast care, breast-feeding techniques, preparation of powdered milk and bottle-feeding techniques, child spacing	At general hospital, no breast-feeding allowed "in order to prevent infection"; at maternity clinic, 24 h after delivery	If mother not yet secreting milk at 8 h after delivery, powdered milk given	In maternity clinic, breast-feeding encouraged	as above	as above
Hungary	all	obstetrician paediatrician midwife nurse	Breast care, breast-feeding techniques	12–24 h after delivery	Fixed schedule: every 3 h until infant reaches 4 kg, then every 4 h	Specially trained staff encourage breast-feeding		
Sweden	all	nursery nurses nurse assistant nurse special instructor	Breast-feeding discussed with all mothers immediately after delivery	2–6 h after delivery; recently, immediately after delivery (5–15 min) for some mothers	A slightly flexible schedule (about every 4 h); in rooming-in, the trend is towards feeding on demand	Breast-feeding considered normal feeding method and encouraged by staff		

[a] See footnote to Table 1.

Table 39. Postnatal services

Country	Group[a]	Location	Personnel	Services
Ethiopia	A	hospital private clinics	obstetrician paediatrician midwife nurse	Physical examination, advice on infant nutrition, especially breast-feeding; immunization; irregular visits until child 5 years old; high drop-out rate
	C	municipal clinic	health officer midwife nurse health assistant	as above
	R	health centre	community nurse health officer traditional midwife	No formal programme; health centre with limited service 50 km away
Nigeria	R	teaching hospital general hospital general practitioner hospital maternal and child health centre maternity centre	obstetrician paediatrician physician midwife nurse auxiliary nurse	Weighing, examination, demonstration of weaning food preparation, child care, immunization, and family planning; regular visits during first 8 weeks, then variable; mothers encouraged to attend weekly clinics
Zaire	all	paediatric services in hospital health centre	physician nurse auxiliary nurse	7–8 visits during first 2 years

Chile	A	private clinics	obstetrician paediatrician	Usually 2 visits in first month, monthly visits during first year and 3 visits during second year; immunization
	C	outpatient clinics	obstetrician paediatrician nurse/midwife auxiliary nurse	Regular check-up from birth to 6 years; physical examination, advice on infant nutrition, especially breast-feeding, and on food supplementation; immunization
	R	rural hospital outpatient clinics	as above	as above
Guatemala	A	private clinics	obstetrician paediatrician	Monthly visits during first year, and 4 visits during the second year
	C	hospital	obstetrician and paediatric residents physician	Advice on infant nutrition, especially breast-feeding, immunization, anthropometry; one visit per month advised
	R	health centres domiciliary	physician midwife auxiliary nurse traditional midwife	as above
India	A	hospital clinic	obstetrician paediatrician neonatologist health visitor public health nurse	Advice on infant nutrition, especially breast-feeding, immunization, child guidance clinics for problem children in special centres; mothers advised to bring infants for monthly check-ups, but rarely do, except in some urban centres catering for an elite

Table 39 (*contd*)

Country	Group[a]	Location	Personnel	Services
India (*contd*)	C	hospital maternal and child health centre	obstetrician paediatrician neonatologist public health nurse health visitor auxiliary nurse/midwife health educator	as above
	R	primary health care centre hospital (depending on availability)	medical officer public health nurse health visitor auxiliary nurse/midwife traditional midwife	Advice on infant nutrition and care, immunization; mothers advised to bring infants for monthly check-ups
Philippines	A	hospital private clinic	obstetrician paediatrician midwife nurse auxiliary nurse	Paediatrician examines infant at 1 month, then at regular intervals; advice on infant nutrition; immunization
	C	maternity clinic health centre domiciliary	as above	
	R	health centre domiciliary	health officer public health midwife public health nurse auxiliary nurse	Public health nurse visits home once during first week; mother encouraged to visit health centre

Hungary	all	advisory dispensary	obstetrician paediatrician health visitor	Regular check-ups until the age of 6 years; physical examination, review of mental condition, screening tests for tuberculosis, luxation of hip, etc,; infant care and feeding, immunization; vitamins and medicines supplied
Sweden	all	maternity care centres child health centres	obstetrician paediatrician midwife paediatric nurse	Postnatal child health care services: 2 weeks – weight check at centre 6 weeks – first examination 3, 4, 5, and 6 months – examination and DPT vaccination 8, 9 months – examination and polio vaccination 12 months – optional examination 18 months – examination and polio vaccination $2\frac{1}{2}$, 3, and 4 years – examination $5\frac{1}{2}$ years – examination and polio vaccination

[a] See footnote to Table 1.

Table 40. Policy practice concerning premature babies, low-birth-weight (LBW) babies, and babies at risk

Country	Group[a]	Services	Where infant is kept	Feeding policy and practice	Special measures to ensure continued lactation	Mothers' access to and contact with baby
Ethiopia	A	One hospital in Addis Ababa, very few provincial hospitals	In special unit	Mother's milk, otherwise powdered milk	Continual milk expression encouraged	Mothers may stay in hospital as long as required
	C	Patients have to be referred to hospital by municipal clinic (free of charge)	as above	as above	as above	as above
Nigeria	A	Ibadan teaching hospital and one general hospital	Usually beside mother; otherwise in incubator	Mothers' milk if possible; pooled breast-milk used in teaching hospital; otherwise powdered milk	If breast-feeding not possible, continual milk expression encouraged	Mothers encouraged to stay in hospital and be with infant at any time
	C	as above	as above	as above	as above	as above
Zaire	urban	hospital	In special units	LBW babies and babies-at-risk are fed expressed mother's milk, prematures powdered milk	In the case of prematures, mother's milk expressed but not used	Mothers stay in a common room next to nursery
	rural	hospital health centre	At health centre, in heated blankets		If own infant cannot be breast-fed, mother's milk used for other infants	

Chile	A	private clinic	Varies between clinics	Powdered milk and glucose	Little encouragement to continue breast-feeding	Minimal contact, except when breast-feeding
	C	hospital	Special units in all main hospitals	Powdered milk in some hospitals, in others breast-feeding increasingly advocated	Continual milk expression encouraged	as above
Guatemala	A	private hospital	In special unit	Powdered milk	Breast-feeding not encouraged	Minimal contact
	C	hospital	as above	Powdered milk, colostrum occasionally given	Continual milk expression recommended	as above
	R	hospital	as above	Powdered milk	No breast-feeding	as above
India	A	hospital	In special unit	Breast-feeding if possible; otherwise mother's milk given by bottle, or powdered milk	Mothers may remain in hospital to continue breast-feeding	Mothers may stay in hospital to breast-feed
	C	as above	as above	as above	as above	as above
	R	district hospital (if referred)	as above	as above	as above	as above
Philippines	A	hospital	In special unit	Tube- or bottle-feeding; mother's or pooled breast-milk rarely used		If mother wants to breast-feed, infant is brought to her, otherwise no contact
	C	maternity clinic	LBW babies referred to general hospital; heavier infants kept in improvised incubator in nursery	Breast-feeding for heavier prematures, otherwise powdered milk	Continual milk expression recommended	Contact with baby encouraged

Table 40 (*contd*)

Country	Group[a]	Services	Where infant is kept	Feeding policy and practice	Special measures to ensure continued lactation	Mothers' access to and contract with baby
Philippines (*contd*)	R	Usually domiciliary or where patient can pay referred to local medical centre	In improvised incubator	1st day, plain boiled water; baby put to breast when mother starts lactating	Breast-feeding encouraged; otherwise continual milk expression recommended	Mother encouraged to serve as nurse
Hungary	all	hospital	In special unit	Mother's milk or pooled breast-milk	Mothers can stay in hospital to breast-feed or express milk; or breast-milk can be left at the nearest health centre for collection or brought to the hospital	Mothers may stay - in hospital, otherwise regular visits encouraged
Sweden	all	hospital	In special unit	Expressed mother's milk	Continual milk expression encouraged	Parents have daily access; tactile contact in incubator encouraged

[a] See footnote to Table 1.

The practice of using maternal milk for LBW infants seemed to be quite well established. Whether the milk was pooled or whether it was the individual mother's milk depended on the hospital; but, on the whole, there appeared to be a preference for using the individual mother's milk.

Policies with respect to mothers' access to, and contact with, their premature or LBW infants followed no consistent pattern, but for the most part mothers seemed to be encouraged to stay in or near the hospital and maintain close contact with the babies. The extent to which this was possible on a regular basis depended, among other things, upon the nature of the hospital's facilities, the health of the child, and whether the mother was able to stay.

In most countries (except in Chile and among the upper-income groups in the Philippines), attempts were routinely made by hospital staff to encourage mothers who had to interrupt breast-feeding to maintain lactation either by manual expression of milk or by the use of a pump.

When infants needed to be hospitalized, the practice in almost all the nine countries was to encourage mothers to continue breast-feeding them in hospital. In the larger government hospitals serving the urban-poor and rural populations in the Philippines and Chile, as well as in Hungary, there appeared, however, to be few if any facilities for "rooming-in" by the mother.

Maternity leave and benefits

Although legislation covering maternity leave and benefits exists in all nine countries, only in Sweden and Hungary, and to a lesser extent in Chile, was there universal coverage by such legislation. Conditions in other countries were such that only a small percentage of women were eligible to benefit from it. Rural and urban-poor mothers engaged in farm work or in small-scale ventures offering little regular employment seemed unlikely to benefit from maternity protection in many of the countries studied.

From Table 41, which shows the position regarding maternity leave and maternity benefits in the nine countries, it can be seen that there is little uniformity with respect to the type and extent of the benefits provided. The total duration of maternity leave was 6 weeks in the Philippines, 18 weeks in Chile, 20 weeks in Hungary, and 30 weeks in Sweden.

Security of job tenure during post-partum leave was guaranteed in all nine countries, although, as indicated above, the amount of leave to which mothers were entitled varied from one country to another. In Hungary, where benefits are broad in scope, mothers could, in principle, take up to three years' leave.

Day-care and nursing breaks

Provisions for day-care facilities and breast-feeding breaks in industrial establishments were also relatively common in all countries, but the

Table 41. Legislation relating to maternity and maternity leave

Country	Maternity leave	Social security	Allowances	Job tenure during maternity leave
Ethiopia	45 consecutive days of paid maternity leave commencing after delivery; prenatal leave with full pay granted on basis of medical certificate; pregnant women are also entitled to paid leave for check-ups and additional sick leave in case of illness	No specific legislation other than collective agreements between labour unions and management regarding food supplementation programmes in certain industrial sectors		
Nigeria	6 weeks before delivery and 6 weeks after for women in government offices and factories; full pay, if no leave has been taken during year; half pay otherwise No legislation covering privately employed workers, although some firms make their own provisions for employees			Job tenure guaranteed
Zaire	14 consecutive weeks, with at least 6 weeks following delivery; during this period, mother entitled to 2/3 of her salary and continuation of all benefits		Minimum family allowances have been established	Job tenure guaranteed
Chile	6 weeks before delivery, 12 weeks thereafter; women prohibited to work during this period; leave fully paid	Pregnant women and babies aged up to 6 months have right to coverage by National Health Service	Women workers receive $5 per month from 1st month of pregnancy; wives of workers and indigent workers receive a family allowance	Jobs must be reserved

Guatemala	75 days with full salary for women who work for the government and for large industries; majority of mothers not covered for benefits	Paid maternity leave covered by contributions from social security system (2/3) and the employer (1/3)		Job tenure guaranteed
India	6 weeks before delivery and 6 weeks after, provided that weekly contributions have been paid for not less than 13 weeks; 6 weeks leave in case of miscarriage; an additional month's leave for illness, premature delivery, or miscarriage (no employer may knowingly employ a women during 6 weeks following delivery or miscarriage)	Sickness, dependent's, and disablement benefits		Job tenure guaranteed
	12 weeks of leave with benefits if woman has worked for a period of not less than 160 days in the 12 months preceding delivery; an additional month's leave with wages for illness arising out of pregnancy	A woman is entitled to a medical bonus of Rs 25 (US$ 3), if no prenatal care is provided free by employer		Job tenure guaranteed
	90 days at full salary in central government institutions 2 months with pay for permanent government employees			Job tenure guaranteed

Table 41 (*contd*)

Country	Maternity leave	Social security	Allowances	Job tenure during maternity leave
Philippines	2 weeks before delivery, 4 weeks after, on full pay; benefits limited to first 4 deliveries; further post-delivery leave due to illness paid from unused vacation and/or sick credits or allowed without pay	Medical (including hospitalization), disability, death, and retirement benefits	Increases as of May 1977	Job tenure guaranteed
Hungary	20 weeks, usually 4 weeks before, and 16 weeks after, delivery; leave fully paid	Following maternity leave, mother may remain away from work for up to 3 years and get child allowance	Maternity allowance, 2500 Ft (US$120) Child care allowance: 1st child, 800 Ft ($40) 2nd child, 900 Ft ($45) 3rd child, 1000 Ft ($50)	Under the Labour Code it is forbidden to dismiss pregnant or breast-feeding women
Sweden	210 days' leave to be shared between parents; before delivery only the mother has right to this leave, which may be taken 60 days before the presumed date of delivery; in general the maternity/paternity leave money is related to the income up to a certain level, the minimum being Kr 25 (about US$ 5.50) per day		After first 3 months and until child is 16 years old, Kr 1800 (US $400) a year	Job tenure guaranteed

minimum number of women employees needed for day-care facilities to be required varied from country to country. In the Philippines, establishments employing 15 or more "married" women workers were required to provide adequate facilities for breast-feeding close to the mother's place of work; in Chile the minimum number of female employees needed was 20, and in India it was 50.

In India and the Philippines, the law required that qualified health staff should be available to supervise children in day-care facilities, while in Hungary, where large farming "units" and industrial firms were required to provide day-care programmes, it was similarly specified that these should be run by qualified health staff.

There was no uniform pattern with respect to the amount of time allowed for breast-feeding breaks. In Chile, it was up to 1 hour per day. In India, two nursing breaks of 15 minutes were allowed each day, in addition to other regular breaks; these could be taken until the child was 15 months old. Mothers in Hungary were permitted daily breaks of up to $1\frac{1}{2}$ hours for the first 6 months of the infant's life, and of three-quarters of an hour thereafter until the child was 10 months old.

National policies on breast-feeding

In Chile, Nigeria, the Philippines, and Sweden, national policies on breast-feeding and its promotion have been established.

In Chile, the Ministry of Health sponsored a series of "breast-feeding days" which were organized on a regional basis and involved relatively intensive educational and promotional activities. Similarly in the Philippines, the Government set aside certain times during the year for the promotion of breast-feeding, making widespread use of the mass media. A wide range of educational activities to promote awareness of the benefits of breast-feeding has been organized on a regular basis in Sweden, through the press, television, and the health services.

Summary of findings

The part played by prenatal services in preparation for breast-feeding and education on the subject varied considerably; within some groups, these were left to the discretion of staff in attendance. Greater emphasis seemed to be placed on infant feeding in services used by the urban-poor and rural populations.

There was also considerable variation with respect to the timing of the first breast-feed and "rooming-in", the practice of the latter being in no small part determined by availability of facilities.

The use of mother's milk for feeding LBW infants was found to be common, but policies concerning mothers' access to, and continued contact with, their babies again showed no uniform pattern.

As far as maternity leave, day-care, and breaks for breast-feeding were concerned, it would seem that, although many countries had adopted legislation on these subjects, the extent to which mothers were covered by it varied extensively. The existence of such legislation should not be taken *ipso facto* to mean that maternity leave and maternity benefits are being enjoyed by all mothers. In many cases, vulnerable women in poor urban and rural communities have the wrong type of employment to qualify for them, and thus benefit the least.

There has been little interest in establishing national policies on breast-feeding. This may reflect limited concern about infant nutrition and the steps that should be taken to promote better infant-feeding practices.

10. Marketing and distribution of breast-milk substitutes

The survey on the marketing of breast-milk substitutes in developing countries described in this chapter was complementary to the collaborative studies on breast-feeding reported in the preceding chapters. The infant-food market in those countries is to a large extent supplied by transnational companies based in Asia, Europe, and the USA. The survey had, therefore, to cover the marketing policy of companies at the headquarters level and its effect in individual developing countries.

The four countries selected were Ethiopia, India, Nigeria, and the Philippines. The survey concentrated on producers and distributors of milk products (especially infant formulas) that are designed to replace maternal milk (breast-milk substitutes) or may be so used.

The survey was made in two parts: (1) interviews with headquarters representatives in the home countries of 15 major manufacturers in Europe and the USA; and (2) a field survey in Ethiopia, India, Nigeria, and the Philippines by means of interviews (215 in all) with subsidiaries or country agents of transnationals, local producers of infant foods, distributors, representatives of the mass media, advertising agencies, and marketing agencies, public health personnel and administrators, and (for "shelf studies") owners or managers of retail establishments. These interviews were carried out between April 1976 and May 1977, and the information given in this chapter relates to that period, except for some retrospective data.

Infant-food companies

Marketing practices

All the companies studied were active in developing countries; between them they produced 50 different brand products and 200 varieties of infant foods. Each was represented in between 50 and 100 countries, and about half of them had established factories in developing countries; most of them also had subsidiaries throughout the Third World.

The distribution networks used by these industries included pharmacies, food stores, and other commercial outlets. Almost all of them also worked, in one way or other, through the health sector, which in some cases meant regular visits on the part of salesmen to health care institutions and to health personnel. Some companies also employed "nurses" or "mothercraft" staff working within, or having access to, health institutions and the mothers attending them.

The distribution of free samples was a relatively common practice, although it varied considerably in scale according to the company and the national setting; about half the companies reported that they also distributed free bottles to hospitals and as gifts to mothers.

For the most part, the products being marketed were felt to be aimed at the more affluent sections of the market, but it appeared that most companies had not established clear target groups for their marketing programmes and were thus not sure to whom their products were eventually going. Budgets were sometimes allocated for advertising in individual countries, the responsibility for promotion and distribution being handed over to independent groups in these countries.

Decision-making structures

Many of the companies covered by the study were parts of large conglomerates, and it was often difficult to obtain a complete picture of their structures. It was evident, however, that, although many of them followed different forms of organization, marketing divisions and departments responsible for sales to and within developing countries were well established parts of all the companies.

Most companies indicated that they saw themselves as relatively centralized, but that the degree of centralization varied according to the type and sphere of operation. For example, product formulation, packaging, branding, pricing, promotional activities, product positioning, and the development of targets for market growth were all felt to be highly centralized and standardized activities. Decisions concerning market segmentation and choice of distribution channels for products, on the other hand, were relatively decentralized and were in some countries handed over to independent groups.

Policy questions

There was little evidence that companies had developed any policies on market limitation, market growth, or market segmentation, or that they had recognized that different population groups have different types of needs.

While many of the companies had independently established or subscribed to codes of marketing conduct, these were often guidelines for marketing rather than expressions of fundamental business philosophies. For the most part, industry appeared to be product-oriented and primarily concerned with supplying the best possible infant-food product with the best possible instructions to existing natural markets, which they perceived as growing of their own accord. Most of the companies indicated that they fulfilled a basic need and did not feel it necessarily their responsibility to restrict their activities or to ensure that mothers who could adequately breast-feed did not buy their products. Few companies had undertaken studies of the possible adverse effects of bottle-feeding, and no company reported an established system for monitoring or carrying out research on them.

Country surveys

Type and size of markets

A total of 42 transnational companies from 13 countries were found to be marketing milk products in the four survey areas. The extent of their presence varied considerably; in India, for example, there were 3 transnational or affiliated companies, while in Ethiopia there were 24. Some of the companies limited their activities to the production and marketing of foods; others were involved primarily in the production and marketing of pharmaceutical products, with infant foods as a sideline.

In Ethiopia, Nigeria, and the Philippines, the breast-milk substitute market was almost entirely supplied from abroad, products being imported already packaged or in bulk form ready for local packaging. In India, where there was some local production, transnational subsidiaries nevertheless exercised a strong influence.

Table 42. Number of different types of milk product found in survey areas

Country	Infant formulas	Other milk-based products	Condensed or evaporated milk	Total
Ethiopia	23	15	8	46
Nigeria	20	14	7	41
India	8	8	4	20
Philippines	24	22	12	58

As can be seen from Table 42, a large number of infant formulas and other milk products that could be used as breast-milk substitutes were being marketed. The smallest number of brand products found being marketed in any one survey area was 20 in India. In the other countries, the number of products varied between about 40 and 60. In some of the markets studied, milk powder and condensed milk products were often accompanied by bottle-feeding tables suggesting that they were intended to be sold as infant foods.

Brand products usually came in several forms, often involving different product formulations and package sizes; when all the variations are taken into account, the total number of products on the market in any one country could amount to 2–3 times the number of brand names.

As far as infant formulas are concerned, the number of products being marketed ranged between 8 in India and 24 in the Philippines.

Sales volume

The absence of proper definitions for products and the general lack of reliable statistics made it difficult to calculate the exact volume of milk products supplied to the different markets through either private or public distributors. The figures summarized in Table 43 are thus estimates based on calculations made by respondents. The total amount of infant formulas sold in the four countries during 1975–76 was approximately 37 000 t with an overall sales value of US $123 million.

Table 43. Estimated annual sales volume and market value of different types of milk product, 1975–1976

Country	Infant formulas		Other milk-based products		Condensed or evaporated milk	
	sales volume	market value	sales volume	market value	sales volume	market value
	t	US$ (millions)	t	US$ (millions)	t	US$ (millions)
Ethiopia	300	1.3	600	2.4	100	0.1
Nigeria	10 000	48.3	8 000	35.3	35 000	56.4
India	20 000	51.0	8 000	19.5		
Philippines	7 000	22.2	4 500	11.2	68 000	56.3

Among the four countries, India constituted the largest market, followed by Nigeria and the Philippines. In the two latter countries, sales of condensed milk were also significant. The extent of the inroads made by commercially prepared foods in these national markets can be estimated by relating the volume of sales reported to the number of potential consumers. Table 44, for example, shows the amount of products sold per baby born in 1975 and suggests that the marketing of such foods in Nigeria and the Philippines, where over 3 kg of infant formulas were sold per baby as against less than 1 kg in Ethiopia and India, was considerably more effective than in the latter countries.

Prices and estimated purchasing power

The price of products relative to earning power was estimated by comparing the estimated cost of 6 months' full feeding using infant

Table 44. Annual sales of different types of milk product, by weight, 1975–1976, per baby born in 1975*

Country	No. of births	Infant formulas sold	Other milk-based products sold	Condensed or evaporated milk sold
	millions	kg	kg	kg
Ethiopia	1.4	0.2	0.4	0.1
Nigeria	3.1	3.2	2.6	18.0
India	24.5	0.8	0.3	
Philippines	1.9	3.6	2.3	35.0

* Population data from Population Reference Bureau Inc: *1975 World population data sheet.*

formulas with personal income over a similar period. As can be seen from Table 45, in all four countries the cost in relation to the average income was high. In Ethiopia, for example, to feed an infant over a 6 month period, using the most expensive formula available in that country, would cost more than the country's *per capita* gross national product (GNP), and certainly more than the income of those who are not part of the cash economy.

Table 45. Cost of feeding an infant with an infant formula for 6 months*

Country	*Per capita* GNP, 1975	Cost of infant formula	
		in US$	as percentage of *per capita* GNP
Ethiopia	100	54–140	50–140
Nigeria	340	60–138	20–40
India	140	51–79	40–60
Philippines	380	49–127	15–30

* Requirements for full feeding over 6 months, calculated according to instruction tables on packages for 6 selected brands, shows an average of 22 kg, equivalent to 3.7 kg/month. The cost is shown as the range between the costs of the lowest and the highest priced products. GNP data from *1975 World Bank Atlas*, Washington, DC, 1976.

Distribution of bottles

In all four countries studied, there was a plentiful supply of feeding-bottles on the market; in some cases infant-food companies also supplied bottles free through health services. Of the 5 million feeding-bottles estimated to be sold or given away in these countries each year, most are imported; only in India was there any significant national production of bottles. In Ethiopia, 9 major brands were identified; in India, 4; in Nigeria, 11; and in the Philippines, 5. Other brands, however, may have existed.

Extent of marketing coverage

Different geographical areas

On the basis of interviews with company representatives and distributors, it appeared that in Ethiopia and India the outreach achieved was scattered and that the main foci for marketing continued to be in the urban areas. In Ethiopia, 90% of the market was reported to be centred in Addis Ababa, and in the Philippines 80% of all infant foods were reportedly sold in the Manila area. In the Philippines, however, there is no specific geographical segmentation and products are sold through a variety of distributors and wholesalers, wherever demand exists. In Nigeria, coverage appeared to be relatively even throughout the country.

Market segmentation

Representatives of infant-food companies at the country level stated that, in all the areas studied, a natural segmentation of the market had emerged and that only those consumers who could genuinely afford the products were being exposed to them and were buying them. However, no data existed to support this statement, and the distributors themselves reported that they were not limiting the distribution of products by either geographical or socioeconomic criteria. The attitude generally expressed by companies was that the market for infant foods would grow as a result of population growth and increasing purchasing power.

Distribution networks

Commercial distribution

Dual distribution systems existed in all four countries studied. Modern westernized systems of distribution, which included food and pharmaceutical retailers and self-service stores, were operating, as well as more traditional channels which included general stores, kiosks, and open market stalls.

In some of the large urban areas, both systems functioned side by side, but, in rural areas, there was usually only the traditional system. In the modern sector where there were large retail chains, these often worked closely with wholesale systems; in the traditional sectors, the marketing network was mainly composed of small-scale independent businessmen who functioned both as wholesalers and as retailers. Companies that made food and pharmaceuticals tended to use large food stores and pharmacies as outlets, while companies producing only food relied more on distribution through networks of small retail stores.

For the most part the infant-food industry worked through large-scale distributors who were both importers and wholesalers and who often entered into agreements on particular merchandise with suppliers. Distributors usually bought a variety of products from different companies and, in turn, sold their products to small-scale wholesalers and retailers. Because of poor transport in many areas, the physical distribution of products was often a problem and control of transport facilities ensured a key position in the market.

Although a relatively large number of infant-food companies was present in all four countries and the variety of brands sold was large, the market nevertheless tended to be dominated by a few large companies. As can be seen from Table 46, the largest of these companies accounted for about 40% of the infant-formula market and the four largest companies together controlled between 90% and 99% of the market.

Table 46. Distribution of the infant-formula market in the survey areas among the four largest companies involved

Country	Estimated share of the market[a]			
	largest company	two largest companies	three largest companies	four largest companies
	%	%	%	%
Ethiopia	40	65	85	95
Nigeria	40	59	77	90
India	63	79	92	95
Philippines	47	85	99	99

[a] According to sales volume by weight.

Public distribution

In most of the countries studied, there was some free distribution of infant foods by both national and international aid organizations; in some cases the foods being distributed were of the type that could be used as breast-milk substitutes. However, there was no indication that feeding-bottles were ever provided as part of the food distribution programmes, nor was there any indication that the products distributed were being presented to mothers as breast-milk substitutes. Distribution was mainly through the public health sector or through specially organized distribution centres, but in some areas it was also carried out through the school system. The outreach achieved by the programmes was often extensive and penetrated into the rural areas.

Marketing practices

Sales through representatives

Sales through representatives' visits were generally felt to be important for market growth in all the countries studied, and elaborate sales organizations had been established; these were based on sales representatives and supervisors, who covered the market through regular visits and whose activities were in turn monitored for productivity by management staff. The principal objective of the sales representatives was to promote their companies' products, and improved sales performances were encouraged through income incentives.

Promotional activities

Table 47 summarizes the different types of promotional activities observed in the four countries. The support cost for these activities usually represented between 1% and 4% of the gross sales of the products involved.

Table 47. Promotional activities by infant-food companies in the survey areas*

	Ethiopia	Nigeria	India	Philippines
Total no. of companies	11	7	5	4
Number of companies using:				
advertising	5	3	5	4
newspapers	2	1	5	4
magazines	1	1	5	4
radio	3	1	3	3
television	3	1	1	3
cinema	0	1	2	0
professional journals	1	3	3	2
sales promotion	11	7	5	4
posters/stickers	8	6	4	4
free samples	8	7	1	3
booklets and pamphlets	6	6	3	3
gifts of various kinds (including bottles)	4	3	0	4
public relations techniques				
sponsoring of conferences	2	5	3	2

* The table relates to 1976–1977 and mainly to infant-formula advertising, although the advertising of milk products with feeding tables has been included. In the Philippines one company did not answer. Two of the companies answering did not sell infant formulas or powdered milk with bottle-feeding labels on the packages and have therefore been excluded.

In all four countries, there appeared to have been some diminution of the amount of mass-media advertising, but, during the period of the study, Nigeria and the Philippines (where *per capita* sales were highest) were still the scene of intensive promotional activities, certainly to a greater extent than India or Ethiopia, where the amount of advertising through the press and radio had been significantly reduced.

In the Philippines, there was also considerable advertising of evaporated milks, milk powder, and feeding-bottles.

Marketing through the health sector

Pharmaceutical companies have traditionally provided physicians and other health personnel with information on their products through personal visits by salesmen. This technique appears to have been adopted by many infant-food companies too, and in Nigeria and the Philippines it was complemented by an active use of "mothercraft nurses" in a health service setting.

Considerable amounts of free infant formulas were also being provided to health institutions, and it was estimated, for example, that the average clinic in Nigeria might receive up to 8000 cans of baby food in the course of a year. Private clinics tended to receive even more than public health institutions. It was estimated that, in Nigeria and the Philippines, up to 1.5 million cans of infant formulas, representing 1% and 7% respectively of the total sales volume in those countries, were provided free. Promotional activities of this type did not appear to be particularly common in either India or Ethiopia.

Retail stores

Table 48 shows the number of brands found on sale in a variety of retail outlets. By far the highest number of varieties of infant formula (54 brand varieties) was found in supermarkets in the Philippines. Small local kiosks and market stalls in the Philippines also offered a relatively broad selection of products, in some cases up to 6 different types. The way in which products were presented often made it difficult to distinguish between those that were meant as breast-milk substitutes and other milk foods. This was particularly so when products such as milk powder and condensed milk were presented in containers that had feeding-tables printed on the labels.

Table 48. Number of brand varieties of infant formulas and other milk products found in different types of retail outlet

Country	No. of brand varieties per type of retail store								
	supermarkets			pharmacies			other stores (kiosks, etc.)		
	infant formulas	other milk products	total	infant formulas	other milk products	total	infant formulas	other milk products	total
Ethiopia	10	12	22	<1	0	<1	2	2	4
Nigeria	10	6	16	7	3	10	5	4	9
India				4	2	6	5	4	9
Philippines	18	36	54	19	9	28	6	6	12

Summary of findings

Multinational infant-food companies were active in the four countries in which the field study was undertaken. Infant foods, including formulas and other products that could be used as breast-milk substitutes, were sold through a wide variety of commercial outlets. Providing free samples was relatively common, although the use of this technique differed in intensity according to the country in question.

Policies concerning the centralization of decision-making varied, but, on the whole, such things as product formulation, packaging, branding, and pricing were centralized activities, while responsibility for market segmentation and choice of distribution channels was decentralized.

Few companies appeared to have undertaken studies or developed mechanisms to monitor the possible adverse effects of bottle-feeding. There was a general belief that natural segmentation would prevent the purchase of certain products by low-income families who could not use them correctly.

The number of products actually being marketed varied considerably and, in many situations, included foods that were not expressly designed as breast-milk substitutes but nevertheless carried feeding-tables on the labels. Sales of condensed milk, for example, were significant in Nigeria and the Philippines.

Some reduction in the intensity of advertising was reported in all four countries, but, in Nigeria and the Philippines, where sales were highest, there was still a considerable amount of advertising through the media and other channels.

Relative to earnings, the cost of infant foods was high, particularly in Ethiopia where it was estimated that feeding an infant for 6 months with the most expensive formula would cost more than the GNP *per capita* for a year.

The geographical extent of the marketing of infant foods, however, varied considerably; in Ethiopia, it was said to be centred on Addis Ababa. In the Philippines, the picture was not entirely clear, since a wide variety of sales outlets was used whenever a demand was felt to exist.

Dual distribution systems were being used in all countries, which meant that products were available through kiosks and market stalls as well as supermarkets and pharmacies. The latter were more often used by companies that produced both pharmaceutical and food products, while companies producing only food worked primarily through small retail stores.

11. Conclusions

This chapter deals with some of the main points raised by the collaborative study, highlights the principal issues, and, it is hoped, provides some guidelines for those responsible for formulating action programmes. It is not a complete summary of the findings—this is provided by the summaries at the end of each chapter.

The aim of the study was to obtain, using standardized methods and centralized analysis, a reliable and objective picture of current infant-feeding practices, with special reference to breast-feeding, in various parts of the world.

In each of the countries included in the study, information was collected by national investigators from families living in economically advantaged urban areas, urban-poor areas, and rural areas with a traditional way of life (questionnaire B in Annex 2). In two countries, middle-income families were also studied.

Information was also collected on health service practices, social legislation, and the marketing of breast-milk substitutes in order to obtain a more complete picture of the possible influence of some of the factors and conditions associated with different feeding practices (questionnaire A in Annex 2).

Statistical considerations

The 25 groups that were studied comprised approximately 23 000 mother/child pairs. They are considered typical of the communities from which they were drawn, though not necessarily representative of the national situation. Comparisons between different groups from the same country are likely to be valid, but comparisons between nominally similar groups in different countries have to be made with caution.

In order to maximize the information obtained for a given effort and to minimize errors due to poor follow-up or faulty recall, a cross-sectional rather than a longitudinal design was chosen. This imposed certain constraints on the interpretation of the data which, it was felt, were more than compensated for by the larger numbers covered and the greater accuracy obtained. Most of the information derived from the study is based on point-prevalence data and thus avoids errors due to faulty recall. With a small number of questions—for example those relating to birth weight—it was necessary to rely on the mother's memory and, in the absence of records against which to verify the answers, the information obtained may be less reliable.

The situations studied were inherently complex, involving large numbers of interacting events. Any straightforward description of the facts, such as that presented in the preceding chapters, is thus a very difficult task, even though each fact may be simple in itself. The main purpose of the present report is to highlight the principal trends and issues involved. An analysis of some aspects in greater depth could be carried out later if desired. As in any study of this nature, it is possible, with hindsight, to single out questions that were ill-adapted or not relevant to given social situations—for example, that relating to employment.

The prevalence and duration of breast-feeding

The patterns of prevalence and duration of breast-feeding varied considerably between countries and population groups. In some groups, all mothers breast-fed for at least one year. At the other extreme, over 30 % of mothers in some groups did not even initiate breast-feeding. Nevertheless three main patterns emerged; in the first, which was labelled Category I, breast-feeding was rarely continued beyond 6 months post partum, and indeed there was a general tendency to terminate it considerably sooner. Most of the mothers in this category came from Hungary and Sweden and from economically advantaged urban communities in other countries.

At the other extreme was Category III, in which breast-feeding was prolonged and almost universal, and in which about half of the mothers were breast-feeding at 18 months post partum. In no group in this category did more than 2 % of mothers fail to initiate breast-feeding. It included most of the urban-poor groups, all the rural ones, and, interestingly, the economically advantaged group in Zaire. Category II, falling midway between the other two, included most other mothers.

It is difficult to explain these variations in breast-feeding on purely biological grounds. Certainly it is interesting to note that the social and economic groups that were less favoured as regards general health, nutrition, and environmental conditions were the very ones in which breast-feeding was most prevalent and prolonged, and presumably most successful. Meanwhile, in the groups more favoured in these respects, the prevalence and duration of breast-feeding were low. This suggests that differences in breast-feeding behaviour are determined by personal preference, conditioned by custom or social and economic circumstances rather than by the biological ability to lactate. It is difficult to believe, for example, that up to 20 % of mothers from economically advantaged backgrounds in Guatemala and the Philippines were—as the data suggest—really unable to breast-feed. It should be possible, by suitable educational and supportive activities, to encourage more mothers from such backgrounds to breast-feed. This does not necessarily mean that *all* mothers could have breast-fed for prolonged periods, but the data do suggest that the proportion of mothers with deficient lactation is small, and that most of them should be able to continue to breast-feed over a period of at least 6 months.

The fact that a large number of mothers said that they did not breast-feed, or stopped breast-feeding, because they had insufficient milk does not contradict this. In some countries, however, there were apparent inconsistencies: for example, in Hungary, about 80% of all mothers had stopped breast-feeding by 6 months post partum and about 70% of these gave "no breast-milk" or "little breast-milk" as reasons. Inadequate milk production by such a high proportion of Hungarian mothers appears unlikely, especially if one considers the situation in some of the rural areas studied. A more likely explanation is that Hungarian mothers had been taught that breast-feeding was not sufficient for a baby of 6 months, which again suggests that one of the keys to good infant feeding is to ensure that all mothers are encouraged to *want* to breast-feed, that they understand the physiology of breast-feeding, and that they are provided with the conditions that facilitate and support breast-feeding.

Among the factors that appeared to be positively associated with breast-feeding were early initiation of breast-feeding and frequent sucking. Mothers in Category III, in which breast-feeding was prolonged, for example, all tended to feed on demand and to suckle frequently; those in Category I, on the other hand, were more likely to feed according to a set routine and less frequently. While, in the absence of quantitative data on milk production, it is impossible to demonstrate directly that frequent suckling is associated with a greater abundance of milk, the information obtained does support the view that frequent feeding on demand stimulates milk production.

In some study groups in which higher education was common, many mothers breast-fed for a shorter time than they said was desirable, and it would be interesting to know why this was so. It is possible that, while many mothers realized that prolonged breast-feeding was desirable and gave a response that they thought would be "satisfactory", they were at the same time exposed to influences, beliefs, and pressures that were not readily compatible with breast-feeding. If this is so, it would be important to identify and define these factors and their interaction in greater detail. It is also noteworthy that the overall majority of mothers said they considered breast-feeding to be superior to bottle-feeding.

Lactation and fertility

The relationship between lactation and fertility is an important public health issue, especially in developing countries where maternal and child mortality associated with high unregulated fertility is a particular problem and where modern family planning methods are not always acceptable or available.

The study findings confirm that breast-feeding is accompanied by a delay in the return of post partum menstruation and, presumably, of fertility. Among non-breast-feeding mothers the percentage of women with return of menstruation at given times post partum was remarkably uniform; 80 % to 100 % were menstruating by 3–4 months post partum. By contrast, the percentage of breast-feeding mothers who were menstruating at 3–4 months post partum ranged from 1 % in rural India to 57 % among the urban economically advantaged group in Ethiopia. The patterns of return of menstruation closely accorded with the three categories of prevalence and duration of breast-feeding. Mothers in Category III, for example, in which there was on-demand and full breast-feeding of high prevalence and long duration, were those with the longest post partum amenorrhoea.

Absence of menstruation alone, however, did not necessarily mean absence of ovulation, and the data show that up to 10 % of the mothers who were pregnant at the time of interview had apparently conceived without previously menstruating. The fact that about 70 % of the pregnant mothers in the urban-poor and rural groups in India who were pregnant were still breast-feeding (and presumably at least as many were breast-feeding when they conceived) emphasizes that, while lactation decreases the probability of ovulation and thus decreases the rate of new conceptions at the community level, from the point of view of the individual it is not a very reliable form of family planning. The need for additional contraceptive measures during lactation is clear.

The use of modern family planning measures seems to be far from uniform, and there are areas where they have made few inroads. In rural Africa, for instance, there was a marked absence of such measures, although it has been suggested that, in particular in Nigeria, abstinence during breast-feeding and other traditional methods are widespread. This contrasts sharply with the situation in Sweden, where most mothers were using contraception, and brings out the fact that there are population groups in which, in the absence of continued prolonged breast-feeding, fertility rates can be expected to increase.

It is also noteworthy that, where oral contraception was common, a sizeable proportion of mothers started using it within 3 months of delivery and while they were breast-feeding, thus exposing their infants to the risk of steroid transfer in breast milk.

Family and maternal characteristics

Of the family characteristics that appeared to be associated with patterns of infant feeding, socioeconomic background was among the most important; but since the term "socioeconomic" encompasses such a variety of factors, it is not easy to determine which are the most significant variables. For example, the educational background of mothers was positively associated in Sweden with the prevalence and duration of breast-feeding and in other countries was negatively associated with them.

There was no evidence that paternal characteristics influenced the pattern of infant feeding, except indirectly through socioeconomic status.

The question whether the mother belonged to an extended or nuclear family seemed to be important in Guatemala, where the role of the extended family in supporting breast-feeding appeared to be quite marked, but in general the nature of the family unit did not appear to be significant. Nor did changes in life style associated with residential mobility seem to affect breast-feeding. Migration history was investigated, but it did not seem to have been influential in determining whether mothers breast-fed, or for how long, although it may be that the question on this issue was not sufficiently sensitive.

In the past, it was believed with some reason that, following the same pattern as other aspects of the reproductive process, the efficiency of human lactation would reach its peak in primiparae at about the age of 20 and slowly decline thereafter. Here again, however, the study did not bring out any consistent pattern. In general, then, the data obtained in the study provide little or no evidence that either age or parity *per se* have an important influence on breast-feeding behaviour. In Chile, among the economically advantaged, the percentages of mothers breast-feeding at 3 months post partum decreased with increasing maternal age, while in Sweden and the A groups in Ethiopia and Guatemala, the opposite tendency was apparent. The possible effects of age may, however, have been obscured by the high correlation between age and parity. In Sweden, for example, the percentages decreased with parity, while in Hungary and the Chilean rural group they increased. Only in Sweden was it possible to distinguish between age and parity, and there the prevalence of breast-feeding at 3 months was higher among mothers with first babies and among older mothers.

There was some indication that previous breast-feeding behaviour was an influence, and that mothers who had breast-fed before were more likely to breast-feed again, a fact that is clearly relevant to decisions on the types of educational inputs needed and the mothers to whom most attention should be directed.

As regards the part played by health services in encouraging breast-feeding, it is significant to note that there was no evidence of an association between frequent attendance at prenatal clinics and a higher prevalence of breast-feeding. On the contrary, in some groups in Ethiopia and India, breast-feeding tended to be less common among the mothers who had received the greatest amount of prenatal care. The inverse association between the amount of prenatal care and breast-feeding could, however, have been due to selection factors in the samples. Moreover, the information available on maternal health during pregnancy, for example, was not comprehensive and did not make it sufficiently clear whether the frequent utilization of prenatal care was associated with ill health in the mother. However, the small number of mothers reporting serious illness during pregnancy suggests that frequent attendance for prenatal care was due not to health problems, but rather to health service practice.

It would seem that prenatal care services directly or indirectly discouraged breast-feeding and that pre-existing attitudes among mothers in the various groups usually remained unaffected by their visits for prenatal care. This would corroborate the information gathered with respect to health service management and the lack of clear policies on the promotion of breast-feeding. This clearly indicates the need for more prenatal education on breast-feeding, and encouragement of the practice, especially among mothers from backgrounds where breast-feeding is not customary.

Breast-feeding also tended to be more common among mothers delivered at home than among those delivered in hospital, but this does not necessarily mean that a hospital confinement *per se* has an adverse effect on breast-feeding, since it was possible that, in communities in which hospital confinements were rare, a high proportion of the mothers delivered in hospital were sick or had sick babies. Just as with prenatal care the suggestion that emerges, however, is that the hospital management of breast-feeding, and support and education to facilitate it, should not be neglected, otherwise breast-feeding may suffer.

Data on the prevalence of "rooming-in" in different countries and groups indicate a great deal of variation and suggest that practices in this respect are influenced by the attitudes of individual doctors and nurses, as well as by overall policy. While the findings were not statistically significant, there was a clear suggestion that, in hospital confinements, "rooming-in" favoured the establishment of breast-feeding. Similarly, the timing of the initiation of breast-feeding consistently appeared to have a bearing on its continuation. In Hungary and Ethiopia, there was a significantly higher prevalence of breast-feeding at given child ages when the babies had been put to the breast within 12 hours of birth rather than later; in other groups, even if the differences were not statistically significant, they nevertheless suggested a similar trend.

The mothers themselves did not consider commitments outside the home as an important factor in their feeding behaviour. It was uncommon for them to say that they had stopped breast-feeding specifically because of the need to return to work; nevetheless the prevalence of breast-feeding, as was to be expected, tended to be lower among those resuming paid employment.

While the study did not set out to measure in any depth the possible connexion between breast-feeding prevalence and the advertising of infant formulas or the distribution of free samples to mothers, it is interesting to note that where the level of such advertising or distribution was high, the prevalence of breast-feeding was low. This was especially so in the urban groups in the Philippines, where free infant food samples were common and the promotion of infant formulas was reported to be extensive, involving wide use of the mass media and personal sales visits. However, the giving of free samples was also common among the rural groups, but this did not appear to have had much effect on breast-feeding behaviour.

Characteristics of the children

The data pointed to a fairly clear relationship between the prevalence of low birth weight and the socioeconomic background of the parents, which is in line with previous findings. Except in the Philippines, however, there was little clear evidence that low birth weight had an adverse effect on breast-feeding.

Nor did the data corroborate claims in the literature that male babies are more likely to be breast-fed than female babies; no such sex differences emerged from the present study.

With respect to weight gains, the data are somewhat limited in that, in many cases, the reliability of the reported birth weight depended on the accuracy of the mother's recall. However, the information that was obtained on urban-poor and rural groups confirms the pattern reported from many developing countries—namely, one of reasonably satisfactory growth (by comparison with WHO reference values) up to about 6 months of age, followed by faltering growth. In Sweden and Hungary, and in all the economically advantaged groups, on the other hand, growth was satisfactory throughout the age range investigated, and in the Chilean urban-poor and rural groups, in which the prevalence of breast-feeding was comparatively low, it was also well maintained up to almost the end of the first year. Average weights in India, on the other hand, were substandard even during the first 6 months in all groups; faltering growth was particularly marked after about 6 months in the urban-poor and rural groups.

The study brought out the importance of sound and appropriate supplementary feeding, showing that, in the absence of additional foods by 6 months, there may be some degree of impairment of growth.

The data tend to agree with previous findings of a correlation between high infant mortality and high fertility and an inverse correlation between mortality rates and socioeconomic background. High loss rates among previous children were reported in most urban-poor and rural groups. Without more information on ages and causes of death, this finding can only be interpreted as a general sign of the vulnerability of these groups.

Death rates among previous children of mothers in the urban-poor and rural groups were remarkably high; for example, rural mothers in Ethiopia and Zaire reported no less than 32 % of their previous babies as having died. In general, the rates tended to be highest in the groups with the highest prevalence and longest duration of breast-feeding, presumably because both factors were correlated with poor socioeconomic conditions. This relationship carries with it a warning of the further threat, in terms of both increased fertility and higher infant mortality, that a decline in breast-feeding would pose under similar conditions.

Supplementary feeding

In most countries or groups included in the study, regular supplements were being given to one-third or more of all infants by the age of 3 months, and to more than half of them by the age of 6–7 months. By the end of the first year, regular supplementation was virtually universal, although 15–40 % of babies in poor groups of India and Ethiopia still did not receive it.

Unfortunately, interpretation of the data is limited by the absence of information on the quantities of supplementary foods regularly given, but in general it appears that infants in groups with very low rates of timely supplementation, such as the urban-poor and rural groups in India, showed notably poor growth curves. While it is not possible to show a direct association between late supplementation and poor growth on the basis of the existing data, such an association is highly likely. This is not to say that poor growth rates in older babies may not also be due to infections and other illnesses, but rather that malnutrition and infection may have a synergistic action.

A variety of foods were used as supplements but in general most breast-fed babies given supplements within 3 months of birth received milk or milk-based foods. The use of cereal supplements was more widespread among urban-poor and rural families than among the economically advantaged. Animal products other than milk were rarely given during the first 3 months or, in the case of India and the African countries, even at 4–6 months. Indeed, in the urban and rural groups of India they were not even common during the second year.

Information on the factors motivating mothers to supplement their babies' diets shows that there is a widespread knowledge that babies need supplements, although it is not clear to what extent this reflects concerned awareness of the individual baby's needs rather than a general acquaintance with local beliefs and practices.

There was also widespread awareness of the brand names of the commercial milk-based formulas being sold in all the areas (except in Africa among some of the poor groups), and, while this was more pronounced among mothers who were not breast-feeding than among those who were, the differences between the two groups in this respect were not as marked as might have been expected. There seemed to be no relationship between this awareness and the educational background of the mother, which suggests that marketing influences have penetrated to all groups in the nine countries included in the study.

Most mothers in Sweden and in the economically advantaged groups in Ethiopia, Nigeria, and Chile who were not breast-feeding, or who were giving supplements as well as breast-feeding, had commercial baby foods in their homes at the time of the interview. Of greater interest, perhaps, is the fact that more than half of the mothers in Sweden, and the well-to-do mothers in Nigeria and Chile, who said they were fully breast-feeding, also had commercial baby foods in the house.

As noted above, the average rates of growth of children in Hungary and Sweden, and in all the economically advantaged groups, were satisfactory. The same countries and groups also had the highest percentages of children receiving supplements and the most varied types of supplementation. The general pattern of growth observed may be due in part to differences in supplementation patterns . There was no evidence, except in the case of Hungary, that breast-fed babies who recieved regular supplementation were heavier at given ages than those who did not, but, in view of the theoretical importance of adequate supplementation after 4–6 months of age, further quantitative study would be desirable.

Health services, social legislation, and health legislation

The role of health workers and health services generally in influencing infant-feeding practices can be considerable. They should therefore be consistently in favour of sound practices and provide support to mothers. In the case of prenatal and maternity services, this is particularly important because for many mothers contact with these services is their first introduction to the health care system and comes at a critical time in their lives.

The data collected indicate that, although in some prenatal, maternity, and postnatal services a point is made of promoting breast-feeding, there is in general a marked lack of specific health policies in this respect. Often the content of such promotional activities as exist appears to be left to the discretion of individual health workers and institutions, and in some cases to representatives of infant food industries who work in or through health services. Such was the case in the Philippines and Nigeria, for example.

While no attempt was made to relate the data on promotional policies with those on the prevalence and duration of breast-feeding, it is noteworthy that in both Hungary and Sweden, where information on these subjects is provided as a regular part of prenatal care, the proportion of mothers initiating breast-feeding was high, indeed considerably higher than in the urban populations of some developing countries. It was also observed that breast-feeding was least frequently established among urban economically advantaged groups in developing countries and that, in the maternity clinics attended by these groups, there is little or no attempt to provide regular instruction on breast-feeding or indeed to encourage it at all.

The information obtained on practices in maternity services suggested that there were often no clear policies concerning techniques to facilitate breast-feeding, such as rooming the baby with the mother so as to stimulate close contact, or concerning feeding on demand. Feeding routines varied considerably, and in some instances education on breast-feeding was either lacking or available only as part of general information that automatically included bottle-feeding as well. The timing of the first breast-feed also varied considerably between and, in some cases, within countries, ranging from 2–3 hours post partum to 24 hours or more.

Where domiciliary delivery was common, there was a tendency for breast-feeding to be initiated within the first 6 hours and certainly no later than 12 hours post partum. The exception was the Philippines, where, even in the case of home confinements assisted by traditional midwives, the practice was to delay breast-feeding for about 24 hours after the birth.

In Zaire, Sweden, Nigeria, India, Hungary, and Ethiopia, mothers were encouraged to continue breast-feeding infants who had to stay in hospital.

In the Philippines, facilities for the mother to stay with the infant were provided in private clinics, but there, as in other types of hospital, breast-feeding was not specifically encouraged. In Chile, where mothers were encouraged to continue breast-feeding their hospitalized infants, the hospitals serving the urban-poor and rural groups had few of the facilities needed to make it actually possible for them to do so.

In all nine countries, there was legislation relating to maternity and maternity leave, but the extent of such leave varied, as did the proportion of mothers eligible for it. In Chile, Hungary, and Sweden, 100 % eligibility was reported, but in other countries it was less than 5 %. In most countries there was also legal provision for day-care or nursery facilities in or near the mother's place of work, but this often depended on the numbers of women employed at the establishment concerned. Breast-feeding breaks of varying lengths of time were also provided by most countries in conjunction with crèches but little is known about the percentage of mothers who actually had access to them, found them convenient and used them.

The data on health services suggest that in general they have given some attention—at one level or another, or at one time or another—to the need to facilitate breast-feeding. The fact that actual practices varied so much between population groups and even within countries, however, is indicative of the need for a much more systematic approach to this issue and for the development and implementation of appropriate health service guidelines.

Marketing and distribution of breast-milk substitutes

The information on the marketing and distribution of breast-milk substitutes was derived from a complementary survey carried out in four countries—Ethiopia, Nigeria, India, and the Philippines. The infant-food market is to a large extent supplied by transnational companies; the survey therefore covered marketing policy at headquarters level, as well as in the individual countries.

Most of the companies included in the survey were parts of larger conglomerates and their organizational structure was often complex and difficult to define. Decisions on such processes as pricing and promotion were generally felt to be the prerogative of headquarters offices, while the choice of distribution and retailing channels was delegated to national or regional branches.

Most of the infant-formula market in the four developing countries studied was supplied from abroad and, while there was some national production in India, transnationals tended to exert a strong influence through subsidiary groups.

Despite widespread concern about the influence and impact of infant-formula promotion, there was little evidence that companies had attempted to identify the social groups which their products or promotion were reaching or that they had seen fit to monitor the ways in which their products were being used and with what effect. It was widely felt, among the companies studied, that their products were aimed at the more affluent sections of the public, and that a natural segmentation occurred which ensured that only those who could afford to purchase the products would do so and use them appropriately. There was little evidence of policies aimed at any future limitation of the market, and in fact there was generally a feeling that it would grow naturally. Relative to average incomes, the prices of products were high in all four countries; in Ethiopia, for example, the cost of feeding an infant over a 6-month period, using the most expensive formula in the correct quantities, would have amounted to more than the *per capita* gross national product for a whole year.

The distribution channels used by companies were such that all levels of society were likely to be reached, the only constraint being that of transport. Pharmacies, supermarkets, groceries, kiosks, market stalls, and the health sector were all, in one way or another, involved in the retail process. As far as promotional activities were concerned, about half the companies used the technique of giving free samples to hospitals and individual mothers as well as visits by salesmen to physicians and health facilities; long customary with pharmaceutical companies, such practices appear to be common with some infant-food companies too. In some cases, this approach was complemented by the use of "mothercraft" nurses.

To what extent promotional activities were being modified in response to criticism is difficult to say. Some respondents felt that they had been considerably reduced, but intensive promotional activities were still being carried on in Guatemala and the Philippines at the time of the survey.

Annex 1

Additional tables

Table A1. Reasons given for not breast-feeding (percentage distribution of answers)*

Country	Group[a]	Number responding	Child		Mother						Medical advice	Other
			in hospital, ill	does not suck, "dislikes"	no milk, insufficient milk	breast and nipple problems	ill	emotional problems, beliefs	work, "too busy"	does not want to		
			%	%	%	%	%	%	%	%		
Chile	A	25	16	12	28	16	12	0	0	4	4	8
	C	27	15	11	52	7	15	0	0	0	0	0
	R	21	43	14	29	10	5	0	0	0	0	0
Guatemala	A	69	6	6	43	9	4	13	0	13	0	7
	C	59	20	10	37	3	2	2	0	3	0	22
India	A	37	8	0	59	0	16	0	0	16	0	2
	B	37	3	3	51	0	38	0	0	0	0	5
Philippines	A	190	8	4	37	13	6	3	15	6	0	7
	C	131	5	8	50	12	6	8	8	2	0	2
	R	51	0	12	39	18	8	12	4	8	0	0
Hungary	all	251	0	0	45	0	14	0	0	0	0	41
Sweden	all	47	17	6	23	23	11	13	0	6	0	0

* "Child in hospital or ill" includes some infants hospitalized because of prematurity. No explanation is available for the high proportion of "other" reasons in the returns from Hungary.

[a] See footnote to Table 1.

Table A2. Percentage of mothers using some form of contraception, by age of child*

Country	Group[a]	Age of index child (months) 0–2	3–5	6–8	9–11	12–14	15–17	18 or more
		%	%	%	%	%	%	%
Ethiopia	A	30 (36)	52 (50)	64 (44)	63 (43)	63 (19)	53 (32)	68 (44)
	C	2 (85)	2 (79)	3 (78)	6 (71)	4 (69)	4 (69)	5 (84)
Nigeria	A	3 (36)	31 (61)	37 (59)	41 (58)			
	B	4 (46)	9 (70)	14 (69)	13 (68)	21 (70)	24 (72)	19 (174)
Zaire	A	10 (73)	8 (75)	13 (74)	14 (72)	11 (71)	10 (73)	7 (145)
	C	8 (74)	1 (73)	4 (73)	3 (75)	1 (74)	1 (74)	3 (153)
Chile	A	40 (50)	69 (72)	78 (72)	83 (65)			
	C	44 (48)	62 (71)	62 (71)	56 (68)			
	R	35 (49)	54 (74)	59 (68)	67 (66)	68 (69)	63 (68)	
Guatemala	A	66 (85)	94 (113)	93 (135)	95 (80)	81 (27)	100 (17)	69 (13)
	C	8 (62)	27 (63)	23 (64)	41 (65)	44 (57)	49 (57)	45 (88)
	R	1 (73)	3 (77)	3 (89)	5 (77)	3 (63)	5 (60)	8 (66)
India	A	27 (97)	57 (118)	73 (103)	79 (89)	71 (111)	83 (77)	79 (150)
	B	27 (97)	48 (122)	45 (111)	48 (128)	52 (107)	63 (95)	66 (158)
	C	8 (96)	12 (113)	15 (123)	9 (103)	12 (113)	6 (87)	14 (154)
	R	3 (143)	5 (195)	2 (146)	3 (164)	4 (216)	5 (98)	6 (214)
Philippines	A	38 (76)	84 (83)	81 (69)	82 (51)	84 (44)	84 (43)	80 (76)
	C	17 (114)	44 (117)	49 (101)	54 (84)	54 (68)	49 (76)	64 (106)
	R	3 (122)	22 (107)	30 (110)	39 (87)	52 (83)	49 (75)	49 (136)
Hungary	All	60(1 193)	81 (1 960)	81 (2 131)	79 (1 928)			
Sweden	All	97 (72)	97 (144)	91 (144)	94 (144)			

* The figures in parentheses indicate the number of mothers questioned; these included pregnant women.
[a] See footnote to Table 1.

Table A3. Characteristics of the sample (percentages)

Country	Group[a]	Age of mother (years)		Education of mother		Occupation of mother		Birth order of index child		Family of nuclear type	Husband unemployed
		<20	30 or more	None	secondary or higher	pro-fessional	skilled	first	fourth or higher		
		%	%	%	%	%	%	%	%	%	%
Ethiopia	A	1	19	2	93	67	9	45	15	57	1
	C	12	22	66	7	0	3	29	40	59	7
	R	2	40	98	0	0	0	12	63	70	17
Nigeria	A	0	40	0	98	82	7	27	27	96	2
	B	1	33	4	76	52	9	23	29	93	4
	C	6	31	76	3	0	1	24	21	65	25
	R	2	51	96	0	0	0	24	25	50	43
Zaire	A	14	22	24	35	6	5	18	49	73	12
	C	8	44	78	1	0	3	11	65	72	37
	R	13	37	86	1	0	0	22	51	81	[b]
Chile	A	1	36	0	100	42	1	40	10	85	2
	C	14	26	4	37	2	6	33	22	49	16
	R	17	30	10	22	1	1	30	38	66	8
Guatemala	A	3	23	0	100	63	0	40	12	78	2
	C	11	30	29	9	1	5	24	39	54	3
	R	13	31	57	1	0	2	20	45	70	0
India	A	2	19	0	99	8	2	35	9	62	0
	B	4	17	8	79	3	5	24	23	65	0
	C	13	34	70	14	0	1	23	44	52	0
	R	9	31	90	3	0	4	26	34	35	0
Philippines	A	5	42	0	98	30	13	27	24	50	2
	C	7	30	0	51	0	8	29	36	46	4
	R	6	40	1	24	2	16	26	41	63	3
Hungary	all	5	21	2	27	16	30	45	5	67	7
Sweden	all	6	23	6	72	22	40	48	4	96	5

[a] See footnote to Table 1.

[b] Because of a misunderstanding, the returns from rural Zaire specified that 63% of husbands were "unemployed". However most of them were assiting their wives in agriculture, and, in the opinion of the Principal Investigator, questions on paid employment were not really applicable.

Table A4. Average weights of children by age (both sexes)*

Country	Group[a]	Weight at birth	Weight (kg) at months: 0	1	2	3	4	5	6	7	8	9	10	11	12–14	15–17	18–20
Ethiopia	A	3.3	3.4	4.6	5.2	6.4	7.4	7.1	7.5	9.2	9.2	9.1	9.3	9.7	10.7	10.9	11.6
	C		3.2	4.1	5.0	5.4	6.0	6.3	6.7	6.9	6.9	7.6	8.1	7.9	8.5	9.0	9.3
	R		3.0		4.5	5.2	5.4	5.8	6.4	6.9	6.9	7.0	7.5	7.2	8.0	8.4	9.1
Nigeria	A	3.3		4.6	5.1	6.3	6.6	7.1	7.9	8.3	9.0	9.1	10.1	9.8			
	B	3.4		4.5	5.1	5.4	5.9	6.1	7.0	7.4	7.8	8.3	8.4	9.4	10.6	11.1	12.6
	C			3.7	4.9	5.5	6.0	6.5	6.4	6.9	6.7	7.6	7.3	7.7	8.2	8.6	9.0
	R			4.1	4.7	5.4	5.9	6.2	6.2	6.9	6.9	7.2	7.7	8.2	8.6	9.5	9.9
Zaire	A	3.3															
	C	3.3															
	R	3.1															
Chile	A	3.3		4.0	5.0	6.0	6.7	7.0	7.6	8.1	8.8	9.5	9.3	9.9			
	C	3.2		3.7	4.8	5.4	6.0	6.8	7.2	7.7	7.9	8.5	8.8	8.8			
	R	3.2		3.8	4.7	5.5	5.9	6.7	7.0	7.4	8.2	8.4	9.0	8.9	9.3	9.9	
Guatemala	A	3.2	3.5	4.3	5.3	6.1	6.8	7.7	8.1	8.2	8.6	8.9	9.2	9.7	10.6	11.2	10.7
	C	3.1	3.4	4.7	5.2	5.7	6.1	6.8	7.0	7.2	7.4	8.1	8.5	8.3	8.9	9.3	9.8
	R	2.9	3.3	4.4	5.0	5.6	6.3	6.5	6.9	7.4	7.4	7.6	7.3	7.6	8.1	8.5	8.9
India	A	3.1	3.3	4.0	4.7	5.8	6.2	6.7	7.6	7.8	8.3	8.8	9.4	9.2	9.7	10.2	10.6
	B	3.0	3.4	3.7	4.7	5.4	5.9	6.5	7.0	7.2	7.4	7.8	8.2	8.4	9.2	9.6	9.9
	C		3.3	3.9	4.5	5.1	5.3	5.5	6.1	6.9	7.1	7.1	7.1	7.4	7.5	8.1	8.3
	R		3.1	3.7	4.3	4.9	5.8	6.1	6.1	6.6	6.7	6.8	7.0	7.4	7.5	8.1	8.1
Philippines	A	3.1	3.9	4.5	5.3	6.8	7.0	7.1	7.6	7.8	8.6	8.7	9.2	9.8	9.9	10.2	10.4
	C	2.9	3.5	4.1	4.9	5.7	6.1	6.5	6.7	7.3	7.1	7.4	7.5	7.6	8.2	8.4	8.9
	R		3.3	4.1	5.0	6.1	6.3	6.7	7.2	7.0	7.6	7.9	8.2	8.2	8.3	8.9	9.2
Hungary	all	3.2		3.9	4.7	5.5	6.2	6.8	7.5	7.9	8.4	8.8	9.2	9.5			
Sweden	all	3.5	3.8	4.7	5.4	6.1	6.7	7.3	7.8	8.4	8.7	9.4	9.6	10.2			

* Birth weights are from retrospective data. Other weights are weights at time of interview.
[a] See footnote to Table 1.

Table A5. Percentage of breast-fed children, by age, who were breast-fed only or given various supplements during week before interview

Country	Group[a]	Type of feeding[b]	Age of child (months)									
			0–1	2–3	4–5	6–7	8–9	10–11	12–13	14–15	16–17	18 or more
			%	%	%	%	%	%	%	%	%	%
Ethiopia	A	(i)	67	18	8							
		(ii)	0	14	0							
		(iii)	0	11	17							
		(iv)	33	57	75							
	C	(i)	90	49	47	61	37	22	13	7	8	12
		(ii)	0	2	2	0	0	0	3	0	0	0
		(iii)	6	16	18	16	27	34	39	33	28	47
		(iv)	4	33	33	23	36	44	46	59	64	41
	R	(i)	78	46	6	15	8	8	5	13	4	1
		(ii)	11	5	0	0	1	2	0	3	0	0
		(iii)	7	18	29	32	41	39	51	34	40	51
		(iv)	4	31	65	53	49	52	43	50	56	48
Nigeria	A	(i)	5	11	4	0						
		(ii)	0	3	0	0						
		(iii)	0	0	0	0						
		(iv)	95	86	96	100						
	B	(i)	4	0	0	0	0	0				
		(ii)	52	2	4	0	0	0				
		(iii)	4	0	0	0	3	15				
		(iv)	40	98	96	100	97	85				
	C	(i)	8	8	0	5	0	0	0	0	0	0
		(ii)	32	29	12	3	4	6	4	2	2	2
		(iii)	0	0	0	2	2	2	2	0	0	0
		(iv)	60	63	88	90	95	92	94	98	98	98

[a] See footnote to Table 1.
[b] (i) breast-fed only. (ii) breast-fed, plus water, juices, or vitamins. (iii) occasional supplementation. (iv) regular supplementation.

Table A5. (*contd*)

Country	Group[a]	Type of feeding	Age of child (months)									
			0–1	2–3	4–5	6–7	8–9	10–11	12–13	14–15	16–17	18 or more
			%	%	%	%	%	%	%	%	%	%
Nigeria (*contd*)	R	(i)	0	3	4	4	0	0	2	0	2	0
		(ii)	73	62	27	10	2	2	0	4	0	1
		(iii)	0	0	0	0	0	0	0	4	0	3
		(iv)	27	35	70	86	98	98	98	92	98	96
Zaire	A	(i)	96	60	22	16	2	12	0	9	6	0
		(ii)	0	2	2	0	0	0	0	3	0	0
		(iii)	2	11	18	22	16	15	10	19	10	0
		(iv)	2	28	57	62	82	73	90	69	84	100
	C	(i)	84	60	21	4	12	9	9	5	0	1
		(ii)	0	4	2	0	0	0	0	0	0	0
		(iii)	4	4	10	13	16	18	17	7	7	4
		(iv)	12	32	67	83	71	73	74	88	93	95
	R	(i)	78	51	44	24	6	4	2	0	0	0
		(ii)	0	0	0	0	0	0	0	0	0	0
		(iii)	2	14	8	4	2	0	0	2	0	0
		(iv)	20	35	48	72	92	96	98	98	100	100
Chile	A	(i)	35	0	0	0						
		(ii)	25	40	17	9						
		(iii)	0	0	0	0						
		(iv)	40	60	83	91						
	C	(i)	36	20	7	0	0	0				
		(ii)	14	21	3	0	0	0				
		(iii)	0	0	0	0	0	0				
		(iv)	50	59	90	100	100	100				
	R	(i)	48	10	6	5	0	0	0	0	0	
		(ii)	17	31	18	0	0	0	0	0	0	
		(iii)	0	3	0	0	0	0	0	0	0	
		(iv)	35	56	76	95	100	100	100	100	100	

			%	%	%	%	%	%	%	%		
Guatemala	A	(i)	12	9								
		(ii)	10	0								
		(iii)	10	0								
		(iv)	68	91								
	C	(i)	23	7	12	6	0	0	0	0	0	0
		(ii)	62	41	42	7	0	0	0	0	0	0
		(iii)	0	0	0	0	0	0	0	0	0	0
		(iv)	15	52	46	87	100	100	100	100	100	100
	R	(i)	72	65	44	22	0	4	0	0	0	0
		(ii)	24	22	17	13	2	2	0	0	0	0
		(iii)	0	2	2	4	2	0	0	0	0	0
		(iv)	4	12	37	62	96	94	100	100	100	100
India	A	(i)	74	48	19	18	10	0	0	12	0	0
		(ii)	0	0	2	0	2	0	0	0	0	0
		(iii)	1	3	4	3	3	0	4	4	0	0
		(iv)	25	49	75	79	85	100	96	88	100	100
	B	(i)	84	69	51	32	20	17	9	8	4	0
		(ii)	0	1	0	0	0	0	0	0	0	0
		(iii)	1	6	8	1	5	2	2	2	0	0
		(iv)	15	24	41	66	75	81	89	90	96	100
	C	(i)	95	93	91	77	74	64	40	41	29	20
		(ii)	0	1	0	1	0	0	0	0	0	0
		(iii)	0	0	4	3	1	5	6	0	0	1
		(iv)	5	6	5	19	25	31	54	59	71	79
	R	(i)	99	98	96	88	75	52	36	16	11	5
		(ii)	0	0	0	0	0	0	0	0	0	0
		(iii)	0	0	2	0	4	2	2	0	6	1
		(iv)	1	2	2	12	21	47	62	84	83	94

[a] See footnote to Table 1.
[b] (i) breast-fed only. (ii) breast-fed, plus water, juices, or vitamins. (iii) occasional supplementation. (iv) regular supplementation.

Table A5. (*contd*)

Country	Group[a]	Type of feeding[b]	Age of child (months)									
			0–1	2–3	4–5	6–7	8–9	10–11	12–13	14–15	16–17	18 or more
			%	%	%	%	%	%	%	%	%	%
Philippines	A	(i)	7	0								
		(ii)	7	15								
		(iii)	45	39								
		(iv)	41	46								
	C	(i)	41	36	8	9	0	0	0	0	0	0
		(ii)	15	28	17	0	4	0	0	0	0	0
		(iii)	11	13	15	9	11	12	0	4	0	2
		(iv)	33	23	60	82	85	88	100	96	100	98
	R	(i)	26	23	25	2	5	3	3	3	0	0
		(ii)	36	35	17	3	0	0	0	0	0	0
		(iii)	6	13	19	18	7	3	10	7	7	2
		(iv)	32	29	39	77	88	94	87	90	93	98
Hungary	all	(i)	12	3	1	0	0	0				
		(ii)	69	50	7	4	3	3				
		(iii)	6	14	30	27	24	31				
		(iv)	13	33	62	69	73	67				
Sweden	all	(i)	54	6	0	0	0					
		(ii)	27	64	6	0	0					
		(iii)	9	4	6	3	8					
		(iv)	10	27	88	97	92					

[a] See footnote to Table 1.
[b] (i) breast-fed only. (ii) breast-fed, plus water, juices, or vitamins. (iii) occasional supplementation. (iv) regular supplementation.

Annex 2
Questionnaires used in the study

QUESTIONNAIRE A

The following general information should be obtained for each population group and assembled as comprehensively as possible in a form suitable for later use as documentation for the report.

I. General characteristics of the population group

1. Describe the general geographical situation (e.g., semi-urban, periurban, urban, rural)

2. Describe the general housing standard (e.g., luxury "western" type, modest apartments or houses, squatter settlements, slum dwellings, overcrowded accommodation, etc.)

3. Describe the general standard of *sanitation* (water facilities, sewage disposal, latrines or toilets, cleanliness of streets, etc.).

4. Describe the general *economic* standard and to what extent cars, bicycles, electricity, TV sets, radios, bathrooms, refrigerators, and telephones are in common use.

5. Describe the general *cultural, religious, and ethnic* characteristics.

6. Describe special *habits and taboos* related to nutrition and to lactation and breast-feeding.

7. Describe the general *family structure* (e.g., generally stable or unstable, monogamous or polygamous, grandparents living with young families) and indicate the size of the average nuclear family.

8. Give the reasons for *migration* in the area (e.g., seasonal work requiring men to leave home for long periods).

Further comments:

II. General educational level

1. Approximate percentage of *illiteracy* among adults (males and females)

2. Approximate percentage of *school-age children attending school*

Further comments:

III. General economic level

1. In rural areas, indicate whether subsistence farming, commercial farming, or a mixture of the two prevails

2. Indicate the main subsistence and commercial crops and the harvest months for each.

	Crops	*Harvest month(s)*
Subsistence		
Commercial		

3. Is there any season when food is usually in short supply ("hungry season")?

4. At the time of the study is food in short supply owing to (*a*) seasonal factors, (*b*) unusually adverse environmental factors such as drought, flooding, pests, etc. or (*c*) a combination of (*a*) and (*b*)?

5. Where there is a cash economy, describe in general terms the main occupations in the area.

6. Indicate the estimated range of monthly incomes (if applicable).

Further comments:

IV. Foods available

Please use the following table to indicate the foods available in the area for consumption by adults.

Foodstuffs	*Types*	*Consumed*		
		daily	*weekly*	*monthly*
cereals				
pulses/legumes				
green vegetables				
root vegetables				
fruit				
milk and other dairy products				
meat				
fish				
eggs				

Further comments:

Specify any foods specially *discouraged* for
pregnant women . . . .
lactating women . . . .
infants. . . . .
Specify any foods specially *encouraged* for
pregnant women . . . .
lactating women . . . .
infants: . . . .

Further comments:

V. Availability and cost of breast-milk substitutes

1. Are breast-milk substitutes (i.e., milk-based formulas for infants aged 0–6 months) available?

2. Is manufactured baby food available and on sale in the area?

3. Where are the products indicated in the answers to questions 1 and 2 available (shops, kiosks, etc.)?

4. Is cow's milk or other animal milk used for infant feeding?

5. If commercial products are used, please record here the brand names and indicate the form in which they are sold (e.g., tinned powered milk, tinned condensed milk).

6. Please calculate the cost per litre (or equivalent) of:
   (*a*) fresh milk;

   (*b*) a frequently used commercial milk-based formula intended for an infant 0–6 months of age.

7. Please indicate what the average weekly income of an unskilled worker (e.g., a farm labourer, office cleaner, or factory hand) is likely to be.

8. How are breast-milk substitutes advertised to the people in the area (e.g., by TV, radio, newspaper, posters, sales campaigns)?

9. Describe the advertising effort made to promote breast-milk substitutes (e.g., very intensive and aggressive, quite intensive, not very intensive, not at all intensive)?

10. Are breast-milk substitutes distributed to families free of charge?

11. If so, where (e.g., at maternity ward or delivery centre, at maternal and child health centre, or somewhere else)? If "somewhere else", describe.

12. What types of children or families, and approximately what percentage of them, would receive free breast-milk substitutes in the area?

13. Are any health-related organizations (local or international) distributing free food in the area?

Further comments:

VI. Working mothers

1. Give a general indication of the extent to which females *work outside* the home (farming, small-scale selling, work in factories or small industries, domestic service).

2. Indicate approximate number of working hours per day (where applicable).

3. Where mothers are actively involved in work outside the home, how and by whom are infants cared for?

4. Describe generally the *domestic work* carried out by females and their workload (fetching water, disposing of sewage, purchasing and preparing food, looking after children, feeding children, cleaning house, getting fuel, etc).

5. To what extent are infants fed by lactating women other than the biological mother?

Further comments:

VII. Maternity leave

1. State whether gainfully employed females are granted maternity leave. If so,

   (*a*) How long?

   (*b*) How much is paid?

   (*c*) Is the law enforced?

Further comments:

VIII. Vital statistics

(If information is not available from official registers, please use data from the sources most closely approximating them.
Please state whether figures are estimated or based on official registers.)

1. Is birth and death registration compulsory? Is it effective?

Birth rate:

Mortality rate, 0–1 year:

1–4 years:

2. Please indicate the most prevalent diseases in the following groups and the seasons in which they occur.

Infants aged 0–1 year:

Preschool children aged 1–4 years:

Adults:

Further comments:

IX. Health services available

1. Describe what type of health service, if any, is available in the area (hospital clinics, etc.)

2. Describe general practices regarding childbirth in the area, including place of delivery (at hospital, maternity clinic, etc. or at home).

3. By whom is the delivery assisted (traditional midwife, health worker, etc).?

4. Length of stay at delivery centre.

5. Describe the maternal and child health activities in the area (percentage of infants and preschool children covered by vaccinations, food and vitamin distribution, etc).

6. Describe family planning activity in the area (organization, acceptance, extent, etc.).

7. Describe infant-feeding practices in the hospitals. Are breast-fed infants kept with their mothers?

8. If the child is admitted to hospital, is breast-feeding continued?

9. Describe in some detail the information, instruction, and recommendations regarding breast-feeding that are given at maternity clinics, maternal and child health units, hospitals, etc.

10. To what extent are the doctors (in particular leading paediatricians and other specialists), nurses, and auxiliaries interested in and informed about breast-feeding, and how actively do they support it?

Further comments:

____

Signature of principal investigator

____

Study Centre

____

Date

QUESTIONNAIRE B

(Reproduction of actual form used)

QUESTIONNAIRE B, PART I	Coding column DO NOT WRITE IN THIS SPACE
0. Card identification B1	1-2: B 1
1. Country	3-4: __ __
2. Area	5-7: __ __ __
3. Family identification number __ __ __ __	8-11: __ __ __ __
4. Name of respondent (mother)	
5. Name of husband	
6. Address	
7. Study Group: urban elite ☐ (1) urban poor ☐ (2) rural ☐ (3) other ☐ (4,5,6) (7,8,9)	12: __
8. Date of interview __ __ / __ __ / __ __ (day month year)	13-18: __ __ / __ __ / __ __
9. Place of interview: Home ☐ (1) Health centre, clinic or similar ☐ (2) Other ☐ (8)	19: __
10. Name of interviewer	
11. Age of mother in years __ __	20-21: __ __
12. Occupation of mother . . . . (1,2,3,4,5 or 8)	22: __
13. Is the mother working this month and receiving pay? Full-time ☐ (1) Part-time ☐ (2) Not at all ☐ (0) Not applicable ☐ (9)	23: __
14. Education of mother:	
a. schooling Yes ☐ (1) No ☐ (0)	24: __
b. number of years of primary schooling ____	25: __
c. number of years of secondary or technical schooling ____	26: __
d. number of years of university or equivalent ____	27: __
e. number of years of schooling outside official school system ____	28-29: __ __
(specify type of schooling . . . .)	30: __
15. Age of husband in years __ __	31-32: __ __
16. Occupation of husband . . . . (1,2,3,4 or 8)	33: __

QUESTIONNAIRE B, PART I	Coding column DO NOT WRITE IN THIS SPACE
17. Is the husband working this month and receiving pay? Full-time ☐ (1) Part-time ☐ (2) Not at all ☐ (0) Not applicable ☐ (9)	34:__
18. Education of husband:	
a. schooling Yes ☐ (1) No ☐ (0)	35:__
b. number of years of primary schooling ____	36:__
c. number of years of secondary or technical schooling ____	37:__
d. number of years of university or equivalent ____	38:__
e. number of years of schooling outside official school system ____	39-40:__ __
(specify type of schooling).	41:__
19. Is the husband now living with the family? permanently ☐ (1) temporarily ☐ (2) not at all ☐ (0) not stated ☐ (7) other ☐ (8) specify.....................	42:__
20. Number of children born alive to mother __ __	43-44:__ __
21. Number of children still living __ __	45-46:__ __
22. a. Age of youngest child in completed months __ __	47-48:__ __
b. age is certain ☐ (1) age is estimated ☐ (2)	49:__
23. Sex of youngest child male ☐ (1) female ☐ (2)	50:__
24. Name of youngest child	
25. Are the mother and child part of nuclear family or part of extended family? nuclear ☐ (1) extended ☐ (2) other ☐ (8) Specify other	51:__
26. How long has the mother lived in present area? less than 3 years ☐ (1) 3 years or more ☐ (2)	52:__
YOUNGEST CHILD	
27. a. Did the mother attend antenatal clinic during the pregnancy? yes ☐ (1) no ☐ (0)	53:__
b. if yes, how many times? __ __ (not applicable 99)	54-55:__ __

QUESTIONNAIRE B, PART I	Coding column DO NOT WRITE IN THIS SPACE
28. Mother's health during the pregnancy:	
generally healthy ☐(1) very seriously ill ☐(2)	
other ☐(8) specify ....not stated ☐(7)	56:__
29. a. Was the mother employed and receiving a salary during the pregnancy?	
yes ☐(1) no ☐(0) does not recall or not stated ☐(7)	57:__
not applicable ☐(9)	
b. if yes, did she receive post-delivery paid leave?	
yes ☐ (1) no ☐(0) not applicable ☐(9)	58:__
c. duration of leave in weeks:______ (not applicable 99)	59-60:__ __
30. Type of birth: single ☐(1) multiple ☐(2)	61:__
31. Weight of youngest child at birth:	
a. _____._____kilograms, not known or not weighed in kilograms ☐ (7777)	62-65:__ __.__ __
b. _____pounds_____ounces, not known or not weighed in pounds and ounces ☐(7777)	66-69:__ __.__ __
32. Present weight:	
a. _____._____kilograms, not weighed in kilograms ☐(7777)	70-73:__.__ __ __
b. _____pounds_____ounces, not weighed in pounds and ounces ☐(7777)	74-77:__ __.__ __
33. Where was the child delivered?	
a. at home unassisted ☐ (1)	
b. at home with unskilled attendant ☐ (2)	
c. at home with traditional attendant ☐ (3)	
d. at home with trained health attendant ☐(4)	
e. at hospital/delivery centre with trained health attendant ☐(5)	
f. other ☐(8)	78:__

TO THE INTERVIEWER:

IF CHILD WAS NOT DELIVERED IN HOSPITAL/DELIVERY CENTRE, GO TO Q. 38

IF CHILD WAS DELIVERED IN HOSPITAL/DELIVERY CENTRE, GO TO Q. 34-37

QUESTIONNAIRE B, PART I	Coding column DO NOT WRITE IN THIS SPACE
0. Card identification B2	1-2: B 2
1. Country	3-4:__ __
2. Area	5-7:__ __ __
3. Family identification number __ __ __ __	8-11:__ __ __ __
34. How long did the mother remain in hospital/delivery centre after delivery? __ __ days, does not recall ☐ (77)	12-13:__ __
35. Was the baby kept in the same room as the mother? yes ☐ (1) no ☐ (0) does not recall or not stated ☐ (7)	14:__
36. Were free milk samples given to the mother in hospital? yes ☐ (1) no ☐ (0) does not recall or not stated ☐ (7)	15:__
37. Was a free feeding bottle given to the mother in hospital? yes ☐ (1) no ☐ (0) does not recall or not stated ☐ (7)	16:__
38. Was the baby given the breast immediately after birth? yes ☐ (1) no ☐ (0) does not recall or not stated ☐ (7)	17:__
39. Is the youngest child breast fed now? yes, by mother ☐ (1) yes, by other ☐ (2) no ☐ (0) if other, specify	18:__
40. If not breast fed now, how long was the child breast fed? breast fed until __ __ completed months of age does not recall, does not know or not stated ☐ (77) never breast fed ☐ (88)	19-20:__ __
IF THE CHILD IS BREAST FED NOW, CONTINUE WITH QUESTION 41 IF THE CHILD IS NOT BREAST FED NOW, GO TO Q. 46	
41. How is the child breast fed? on demand ☐ (1) on schedule ☐ (2) other ☐ (8) not stated ☐ (7)	21:__
42. How many times is the child breast fed during the mother's waking hours? __ __ times, not stated ☐ (77)	22-23:__ __

QUESTIONNAIRE B, PART I	Coding column DO NOT WRITE IN THIS SPACE
43. How many times is the child breast fed during the mother's sleeping hours? ___ ___times, not stated ☐(77)	24-25:__ __
44. If the child is breast fed, what else was given last week?	
a. nothing but breast milk ☐(1)	
b. only breast milk and fruit juice, water and/or vitamins ☐ (2)	
c. breast milk with occasional supplements ☐ (3)	
d. breast milk with supplement every day ☐ (4)	26:__
45. If supplements are given, which of the following were used last week?	
a. milk or milk-based products ☐(1 or 0)	27:__
b. cereals (wheat, corn, rice, sorghum, etc.) ☐ (1 or 0)	28:__
c. animal proteins other than milk (eggs, meat, fish etc.) ☐(1 or 0)	29:__
d. legumes (peas, beans etc.) ☐ (1 or 0)	30:__
e. other vegetables, tubers and/or fruits ☐(1 or 0)	31:__
f. Low cost, protein-rich weaning foods ☐ (1 or 0)	32:__
g. other ☐(8 or 0) specify	33:__
CONTINUE WITH QUESTION 50	
FILL IN QUESTIONS 46-49 FOR CHILDREN THAT ARE <u>NOT</u> BREAST FED NOW, THEN CONTINUE WITH QUESTION 50.	
46. How many times is the child fed during the mother's waking hours? ___ ___times, not stated ☐(77)	34-35:__ __
47. How many times is the child fed during the mother's sleeping hours? ___ ___times, not stated ☐(77)	36-37:__ __

QUESTIONNAIRE B, PART I	Coding column DO NOT WRITE IN THIS SPACE
48. Last week was the child given:	
a. nothing but milk or milk based formula ☐(1)	
b. milk or milk based formula and fruit juice, water and/or vitamins ☐(2)	
c. milk or milk based formula with occasional supplements ☐(3)	
d. milk or milk based formula with supplement every day ☐(4)	
e. no milk or milk based formula given as fluid ☐(5)	38:__
49. Which of the following was the child given last week?	
a. milk or milk based products ☐(1 or 0)	39:__
b. cereals (wheat, corn, rice, sorghum, etc.) ☐(1 or 0)	40:__
c. animal protein other than milk (eggs, meat, fish, etc.) ☐(1 or 0)	41:__
d. legumes (peas, beans, etc.) ☐(1 or 0)	42:__
e. other vegetables, tubers and/or fruits ☐(1 or 0)	43:__
f. low cost, protein-rich weaning foods ☐(1 or 0)	44:__
g. other (specify.............................) ☐(8 or 0)	45:__
50. If milk or milk based formulas are given to the child, how are they given?	
a. by bottle: yes ☐(1) no ☐(0) not applicable ☐(9)	46:__
b. by hand: yes ☐(1) no ☐(0) not applicable ☐(9)	47:__
c. by spoon: yes ☐(1) no ☐(0) not applicable ☐(9)	48:__
d. by cup: yes ☐(1) no ☐(0) not applicable ☐(9)	49:__
51. Is the child using a pacifier? yes ☐(1) no ☐(0) not stated ☐(7)	50:__
52. Does the mother know by brand name any commercial milk based formula?	
yes ☐(1) no ☐(0)	51:__
if yes, specify	

QUESTIONNAIRE B, PART I	Coding column DO NOT WRITE IN THIS SPACE
53. Are there any commercial baby foods in the house now?	
yes ☐ (1) no ☐ (0)	52:__
if yes, specify	
54. How many months after delivery of the last child did the mother have her first menstruation?	
__ __ months	
menstruating, but does not recall ☐ (66) not stated ☐ (77) has not had a menstruation ☐ (88)	53-54:__ __
55. a. Is the mother pregnant now?	
yes ☐ (1) no ☐ (0) does not know ☐ (8) not stated ☐ (7)	55:__
b. if yes, is the pregnancy confirmed?	
yes ☐ (1) no ☐ (0) not applicable ☐ (9)	56:__
56. Is the couple practising family planning?	
yes ☐ (1) no ☐ (0) not stated ☐ (7) not applicable ☐ (9)	57:__
57. If the answer to Q56 is Yes, which method is presently being used?	
a. condom ☐ (1 or 0)	58:__
b. loop (IUCD) ☐ (2 or 0)	59:__
c. diaphragm ☐ (3 or 0)	60:__
d. pill ☐ (4 or 0) specify brand............	61:__
e. foam or jelly ☐ (5 or 0)	62:__
f. rhythm method ☐ (6 or 0)	63:__
g. coitus interruptus ☐ (7 or 0)	64:__
h. other methods ☐ (8 or 0) specify................	65:__
58. If the mother is taking contraceptive pills, how soon after delivery did she start?	
__ __ months; does not recall ☐ (77) not applicable ☐ (99)	66-67:__ __
TO THE INTERVIEWER: PART II the extended interview of the mother is to be:	
filled out ☐ (1) not filled out ☐ (2)	68:__

QUESTIONNAIRE B, PART II	Coding column DO NOT WRITE IN THIS SPACE
0. Card identification B3	1-2: B 3
1. Country	3-4: __ __
2. Area.	5-7: __ __ __
3. Family identification number __ __ __ __	8-11: __ __ __ __
YOUNGEST CHILD	
59. If the mother has never breast fed this child - what is the reason(s)?	12-17: __ __ __ __ __ __
60. If the mother has introduced regular supplementation, how old was the child when she started to do so? __ __ months, does not recall ☐ (77) not applicable ☐ (99)	18-19: __ __
61. If regular supplementation has been introduced, why has the mother done so?	20-25: __ __ __ __ __ __
62. Who or what helped her reach this decision?	26-31: __ __ __ __ __ __
63. If breast feeding has stopped completely, why did the mother stop?	32-37: __ __ __ __ __ __
SECOND YOUNGEST CHILD	
64. a. Age of the second youngest child ____ years ____ months not applicable ☐ (9999)	38-41: __ __ / __ __
b. Age is: certain ☐ (1) estimated ☐ (2) not applicable ☐ (9)	42: __

QUESTIONNAIRE B, PART II	Coding column DO NOT WRITE IN THIS SPACE
65. Have there been any other pregnancies or births between the youngest living child and the second youngest living child? yes ☐ (1) no ☐ (0) does not recall ☐ (7)	43:__
66. How long was the second youngest child completely breast fed? ___ ___ months, does not recall ☐ (77) not applicable ☐ (99)	44-45:__ __
MATERNAL OPINIONS ABOUT BREAST FEEDING	
67. How long does the mother think breast feeding should continue unsupplemented (only breast feeding)? ___ ___ months does not know ☐ (77)	46-47:__ __
68. When does the mother think breast feeding should stop completely? ___ ___ months, does not know ☐ (77)	48-49:__ __
69. In the mother's opinion the child who is between 3-6 months of age will thrive best on: breast ☐ (1) bottle ☐ (2) either equally well ☐ (3) doesn't know ☐ (7)	50:__
70. Was the mother herself breast fed as an infant? yes ☐ (1) no ☐ (0) doesn't know ☐ (7)	51:__
71. If the mother had (has) grown up daughter(s), how long would she advise her(them) to continue breast feeding unsupplemented? ___ ___ months, does not know ☐ (77)	52-53:__ __
72. If the recommendation to daughter is different from the mother's answer to question 67, specify why:..............	54-59:__ __ __ __ __ __
73. When the mother is breast feeding where does she prefer to do it? Only at home, discretely ☐ (1) Only at home, no worry about privacy ☐ (2) Any place, but trying to do so discretely ☐ (3) Any place, no worry about privacy ☐ (4) Not applicable ☐ (9)	60:__

Annex 3

Data collection guides

It is generally acknowledged that the decline in breast-feeding that has been observed in many parts of the world represents a potential danger for the health of infants and that steps need to be taken to halt this decline and encourage more mothers to take up breast-feeding.

Many reasons have been proposed to account for the reported decline. These range from "urbanization" in a broad sense to changes in fashions and norms of modesty that are making breast-feeding less popular and less feasible.

There can, however, be little doubt that the changes that have taken place are multifactoral in origin and that no one single reason for them can be identified. The purpose of this particular set of surveys is to examine three factors: the possible role of health and social legislation in promoting maternity leave and other conditions that facilitate breast-feeding; the extent to which the type of nutrition education given to health and allied personnel is designed to develop their awareness and knowledge of breast-feeding; and the organization of the different categories of health service and how it may influence breast-feeding.

For each of the countries represented in the basic study, it would ideally be valuable to have information reflecting the overall national situation. In the case of social and health legislation this may be feasible, but the surveys on the organization of health services and the training of health-related personnel would, if national in scope, involve far too much data collection. They have accordingly been designed to cover the geographical areas and population groups sampled in the basic study.

To facilitate the collection of appropriate data, the following set of guides has been developed. Within them, series of items are listed which all principal investigators should follow so that the information gathered will be of a standard kind.

It should be borne in mind that these are data collection guides and not questionnaires; that is to say, investigators should feel free to develop items as they see fit and to introduce additional data wherever they feel that this will better explain the situation in a particular country or study area.

Principal investigators may wish to call upon the services of informants or other professional groups who may be more familiar with, for example, the legislative situation. They may also wish to append documents or other materials relating to the issues considered in the survey. This would be entirely acceptable.

It should be noted that, in the case of the surveys on the organization of services and the education of health and health-related personnel, the guides are in two sections: A (general information) and B (more specific data).

NUTRITION EDUCATION IN THE TRAINING OF HEALTH AND ALLIED PERSONNEL

The degree to which health and allied personnel are trained in matters of maternal and infant nutrition may often be the critical factor in determining maternal behaviour with regard to infant feeding.

In particular, such personnel can influence mothers with respect to breast-feeding and the introduction of supplements. In some instances the influential person may be the physician, in others the nurse, the midwife or the traditional birth attendant. In many cases it may be the home economics promoter or the agricultural extension worker in whose routine activities health education is included.

The aim of this survey is to identify the extent to which different categories of health and allied personnel are trained in infant nutrition and, especially, in breast-feeding and are thus able to give mothers suitable information on the feeding of their infants.

The following series of questions, or data items, has been developed as a basis for the investigation. Further items may be added at the investigator's discretion. Investigators should also feel free to go into as much detail as they consider to be needed for as full a picture as possible of how the different laws and regulations of a country might affect pregnant women, mothers of young infants, and the infants themselves.

Investigators should indicate the number of the item or question they are dealing with, as well as any additional information included.

Section A

1. For *each of the areas* included in the basic study, list all the types of health and allied personnel who normally provide services to pregnant women and mothers of newborn infants.

2. Please describe briefly the type of service each of the above might be expected to provide for pregnant women and mothers.

3. Within *each* of the population groups involved in the basic study, which of the personnel listed above is likely to have the most contact with pregnant women and mothers and be in the most influential position to discuss infant nutrition and breast-feeding with mothers?

4. For *each* of the categories of personnel listed above, please complete Section B below.

Section B

1. Please name the category of health worker referred to.

2. Indicate
   (*a*) the type of institution at which this category of worker is usually trained, and

   (*b*) where these institutions are located (with particular reference to the area of the basic study).

3. What is the usual length of basic training for this category of health worker?

4. Are postbasic programmes or refresher courses provided for this category of health worker by the training institutions?

5. Is there a specific course on infant nutrition and breast-feeding in the training programme, or are there more general courses on infant and maternal health that involve information on them? If so, please list them.

6. How many hours of the course are devoted to the subject of infant nutrition and breast-feeding, and what proportion of the overall programme does this represent?

7. Which of the following aspects of breast-feeding are covered in this programme?:
   - physiology of lactation
   - epidemiology of lactation
   - biochemical composition of human milk
   - education for counselling
   - immunological characteristics of human milk
   - influence of maternal nutrition on quality and quantity of breast-milk
   - care of the breasts during the pre-and post-partum period
   - relationship between lactation and ovulation/menstruation
   - relation between lactation and contraception
   - psychological aspects of breast-feeding
   - economic aspects of breast-feeding
   - possible maternal/child health contraindications for breast-feeding
   - health aspects of breast-feeding
   - possible difficulties arising from breast-feeding
   - work, legislation, and breast-feeding.

Indicate the relative importance given to these items.

8. Indicate what teaching materials (texts, papers, slides, etc.) are used in courses dealing with breast-feeding and infant nutrition and, wherever possible, briefly describe the objectives and contents of these courses.

9. Please indicate whether any of the above teaching aids are provided by commercial food companies, health agencies, ministries of health, etc.

10. Indicate whether there is any special policy regarding the ideal age of weaning and the introduction and types of supplementary food.

ORGANIZATION OF HEALTH SERVICES WITH RESPECT TO INFANT NUTRITION AND BREAST-FEEDING

In the same way as health and allied personnel are influential in determining whether and to what extent mothers breast-feed, the organization of the health services helps to determine breast-feeding behaviour. What a mother is told during the prenatal and immediate postnatal period, for example, can be critical in deciding her attitude towards child care and infant nutrition. Likewise the provisions made in hospitals and health centres for encouraging or even facilitating breast-feeding may be of great importance in allowing the mother to establish and continue breast-feeding.

The aim of this survey is to describe the way in which the health services used by the three types of population group covered by the study are organized with respect to breast-feeding and infant nutrition.

The following series of questions, or data items, has been developed as a basis for the investigation. Further items may be added at discretion. Investigators should also feel free to go into as much detail as they consider to be needed for as full a picture as possible of how the different laws and regulations of a country might affect pregnant women, mothers of young infants, and the infants themselves.

Investigators should indicate the number of the item or question they are dealing with, as well as any additional information included.

Section A

1. Indicate, for *each* of the three population groups that were included in the basic study, how the following health services are usually provided:
   - prenatal care
   - maternity care
   - postnatal, maternal, and infant care.

   In particular indicate whether, and to what extent, these services are provided through hospitals, maternal and child health clinics, health centres, domiciliary care, community extension services, etc.

2. Describe the categories of health-related personnel who actively participate in providing these services.

3. In the case of each population group, indicate what percentage of all deliveries is estimated to take place:
   - in hospital
   - in health/maternity centres
   - at home.

4. Indicate whether any food supplementation programmes are currently in operation, and, if so,
   (*a*) how long they have been in operation and how long they will continue;
   (*b*) who runs them;
   (*c*) where they are based;
   (*d*) to whom they are directed (e.g., all mothers, all children, malnourished mothers, malnourished children, all children of poor socioeconomic background, etc.);
   (*e*) the type(s) of foodstuff involved;
   (*f*) the form(s) in which it is supplied, e.g. powder, liquid, solid;
   (*g*) the costs (if any) to the consumer;
   (*h*) whether any educational material or guidance on nutrition is provided through the same programme;
   (*i*) the health or allied personnel involved in providing food supplements.

5. Has there been any pronouncement at a national level concerning the need to promote breast-feeding? Have there been, or are there, any programmes to promote breast-feeding?

6. Indicate
   (*a*) whether the practice of collecting human milk and storing it in "milk banks" is common in the area;
   (*b*) under what circumstances such milk is used.

Section B

B I.

Services provided during the prenatal period, i.e., to pregnant women

1. Describe the types of prenatal service available to the *three population groups* studied and the types of health and allied personnel that operate them.

2. Describe for *each* of the groups and for *each* type of service outlined above:
   (*a*) the place(s) where the services are usually provided;
   (*b*) the number of times that pregnant women would be expected to use these services;
   (*c*) the content (for instance, nutrition counselling and education, child care education, information on breast-feeding and care of breasts) and the information given on nutrition during pregnancy;
   (*d*) the role of the health or allied worker in providing these services.

3. Are there any routine activities within these services that are specifically devoted to education on maternal/infant nutrition and child care, and are demonstration sessions included? If so, please describe them and any teaching aids used in them.

4. Do pregnant women usually receive food supplements through any of these services? If so, please indicate what types of supplement are given and to whom.

B II.

Institution-based services provided to mothers at delivery (not including domiciliary delivery)

1. Describe the usual types of delivery service that are available to, and used by, *each* of the population groups included in the basic study and any differences known to exist in the way the groups use the services.

2. Indicate how accessible these services are to each of the groups and, in general, what the ratio of population to services is.

3. Describe the various types of health and allied workers usually involved in providing these services.

4. Is there a specific policy with respect to encouraging breast-feeding through the maternity service?

5. Describe, giving the reasons for them, the various maternity practices employed (e.g., in hospitals, maternity/health centres, etc.) and, in particular:
   (*a*) the average length of time mothers spend in the maternity ward;
   (*b*) when the child is first given to the mother and put to the breast;
   (*c*) whether the newborn child is kept in the same room as the mother all day and night, all day but not at night, only part of the day, or not at all (if not at all, indicate where newborn are kept).

6. Describe in some detail the feeding routine of normal full-term infants after delivery (for instance, at the breast, with water or sugar water by bottle, with milk formula by bottle, or other routines).

7. Indicate whether infants are fed
   - on demand
   - on schedule
   - other (please specify).

8. Indicate how mothers decide whether to breast-feed.

9. Describe in some detail the information given in the maternity ward to mothers (and fathers) concerning infant feeding. Does it, for example, deal with child-spacing, hygiene, and breast-feeding?

10. Indicate which health personnel usually provide this information.

11. Indicate whether nurses or salesmen representing commercial companies are allowed to go round maternity wards talking to mothers about infant feeding and infant foods. If so, describe the extent and the nature of their activities; for example, during their stay in the maternity service or on leaving it, are mothers given any gifts provided by commercial groups? If so, what are these gifts and to whom are they given (all the mothers or only some of them)?

12. Do the maternity services accept free donations of infant food from commercial companies; if so, indicate which companies and how the food is used or distributed.

13. In the case of mothers who cannot breast-feed (for instance, for medical reasons), indicate what facilities exist for the children to get breast-milk (i.e., wet-nurse, milk bank, etc.).

14. Indicate the approximate percentage of mothers who do not breast-feed at all on discharge from the maternity unit (i.e., whose children are only bottle-fed).

15. What are the policy and practice concerning the care and feeding of low birth-weight babies and other newborn babies at risk? For instance, where are they kept and cared for; what is the mother's access to, and contact with, her baby; what types of food are given; how, and for how long, is the mother's own milk expressed and used for the baby, etc.?

B III.

Domiciliary services provided to mothers at delivery

1. Indicate the overall percentage of deliveries (for *each* of the three population groups) that take place at home.

2. Describe the types of personnel who assist at domiciliary deliveries (for instance, professional midwife/doctor, traditional midwife/birth attendant "grandmother", or similar).

3. Describe in some detail when and how the feeding of the newborn is initiated and how it is continued during the next few days (for instance, when is the child first put to the breast, and later how often; which other foods or drinks are given – what type, when, how often, how much, by bottle/hand/spoon/similar).

4. Describe any special habits/routines relating to breast-feeding and care of the newborn (for instance, whether the child stays close to the mother or not, is separated from rest of family, etc.)

5. Describe in some detail how decisions whether to breast-feed or not are arrived at, and who and what factors are of importance in the decision.

6. Indicate whether, and to what extent, newly delivered mothers are visited by representatives of commercial food companies (nurses or salesmen) and what is the nature of their activities (details of messages, free gifts of baby foods, bottles, and the like, revisits, etc.).

7. Indicate whether any written material about breast-feeding, baby food, or baby care is provided to mothers by commercial companies, government institutions, or other agents. If so, describe the content and types of such material.

8. Indicate whether mothers are followed up by visits at home by a midwife or some other health or allied worker during the neonatal period (about the first month) and, if so, what is the purpose of the visits and the content of the message given at them.

B IV.

Special services for the care of premature and newborn babies at risk

1. Describe what services are available, where these are located with reference to the *three population groups*, and what types of personnel man them.

2. Indicate the frequency of use of these facilities.

3. Indicate whether there is any specific policy or practice with respect to the feeding of premature and newborn babies. In particular, indicate whether maternal milk is used or other pooled breast-milk.

4. Describe the practices followed with regard to allowing or encouraging contact between mothers and babies-at-risk.

5. Indicate any special measures taken to ensure continued lactation in mothers whose babies remain "in care".

B V.

Maternal and child health services provided during the postnatal period

1. Describe
   (*a*) all the services for mothers and children available to *each* of the *three population groups*
   (*b*) the types of health and allied personnel involved in them, and
   (*c*) where and how the services are operated.

2. Indicate the normal routine of visits to mothers and children (e.g., number per month or so), or whether mothers and children come regularly to clinics/health centres etc., and up to what age the child is regularly seen.

3. Describe the content of the services that are *regularly* provided, e.g.:
   – weighing
   – physical examination of mother and child
   – education or follow-up of maternal and infant nutrition
   – encouragement of breast feeding
   – vaccination.

4. If advice on maternal and/or infant nutrition is routinely given, indicate the content of this advice

5. Describe the advice and type of care given to mothers who have breast-feeding problems (either at regular visits or other visits).

6. Indicate whether demonstrations of different methods of preparing baby foods are arranged during visits, and, if so, which types of food (for instance, home-prepared weaning foods, commercial weaning foods, milk formulas, etc.).

7. Indicate whether any checks are made on bottle-feeding (for instance, cleaning of bottles and nipples, dilution of powder, etc.).

8. Indicate
   (*a*) whether baby food is distributed at child health centres and, if so, describe in some detail: type of food; for whom; age when started; amounts given; free/subsidized/full price; regularity of distribution, etc.;
   (*b*) to what extent the distribution is likely to reduce breast-feeding.

9. Indicate whether supplementary foods are given to lactating mothers, and if so, describe the relevant programmes and the types of food provided.

BVI.

Services for infants and children in need of hospitalization

1. Describe the different types and location of the services available e.g., paediatric departments, general hospital, etc.

2. Describe the different types of health personnel involved in the delivery of the services, e.g., doctors, nurses, midwives, specialized personnel.

3. Describe the range of population to which the services normally cater, e.g., high-income or low-income families, etc., and the type of access they have to these services.

4. Indicate the average duration of stay in the services.

5. Indicate
(*a*) whether, when infants are hospitalized, there are any facilities for "rooming-in" of mothers:
– together with children
– separate from, but close to, children;
(*b*) if "rooming-in" is not practised, what are the policies and arrangements for visiting, and what hours are favoured for mothers to visit their children?

6. Describe the policy and practice when children who are being breast-fed are hospitalized, indicating especially whether:
(*a*) they are weaned abruptly regardless of the time they are likely to be hospitalized and, if so, what is substituted for breast milk;
(*b*) weaning is dependent upon the condition and the time they are likely to be hospitalized and, if so, what the usual indications are;
(*c*) the decision is left to the mother and, if so, what advice/encouragement/assistance is given;
(*d*) human milk is used at all in hospital and, if so, whether it is pooled or whether each mother's milk is expressed and specifically kept for her own child.

7. Indicate what the procedure is when, for any reason, the mother's milk cannot be given to the hospitalized infant. Are any measures taken to ensure that lactation continues – for example, by giving the mothers breast-pumps or training them to express the milk manually?

HEALTH AND SOCIAL LEGISLATION AS IT AFFECTS BREAST-FEEDING PRACTICES

The extent to which breast-feeding is practised in a society may, among other things, be related to the provisions made in the country's health and social legislation for such things as maternity leave, maternity benefits, crèches, and nurseries. These amenities or rights often constitute the basis of the support system mothers require if they are to breast-feed their infants.

The aim of this survey is to identify and describe the current legislative situation as it relates to maternity and breast-feeding among the three population groups involved in the basic study.

The following series of questions, or data items, has been developed as a basis for the investigation. Further items may be added at the investigator's discretion. Investigators should also feel free to go into as much detail as they consider necessary to be needed for as full a picture as possible of how the different laws and regulations of a country might affect pregnant women, mothers of young infants, and the infants themselves.

Investigators should indicate the number of the item or question they are dealing with, as well as any additional information included.

1. Describe existing laws in your country on the *working conditions* of women and indicate when they came into effect.

2. Describe any legislation currently in force concerning *maternity* and *maternity leave*, indicating in particular the provisions made in it for such things as:
   - social security
   - maternal leave (fully paid/partially paid; length)
   - family allowances
   - social welfare assistance
   - prenatal and postnatal care
   - food supplementation programmes
   - job tenure during maternity leave.

3. (*a*) What percentage of the female population (of reproductive age) would you say is currently covered by the legislation outlined above? In the case of any exceptions, please indicate whether, and how, any of the criteria listed below are used in defining eligibility:
   - occupational background (e.g., type of job, type of industry)
   - marital status
   - area of residence.

   b. If all women are covered, but variations exist in the *degree* to which they are eligible for different services, please indicate what these variations consist of.

4. Is it known to what extent all industries honour the legislation indicated above, especially as regards maternity leave, job tenure, and any financial contributions they are expected to make? If so, please elaborate.

5. Specify the types of obstacle and resistance that have been met in the implementation of legislation relating to maternity, e.g., from employers or other sources.

6. Is there any legislation specifically providing for:
   (*a*) crèches or day-care nurseries in, or close to, mothers' places of work;
   (*b*) the management of such crèches (if so, indicate where these are usually located);
   (*c*) "breast-feeding" or nursing breaks during normal working hours (if so, indicate the conditions laid down for such breaks)?

7. Where there is legislation on crèches, are the conditions laid down at all dependent on the size or type of the female labour force?

8. Is there any legislation regarding supplementary food allowances (financial or in kind) and, if so, to which groups is such legislation addressed?

9. What mechanisms, if any, exist for enforcing the types of legislation indicated above, and which governmental or nongovernmental bodies are responsible for this task?

10. To what extent would you say the population as a whole is aware of this legislation? Are there, for example, any groups who do not seem to know what provisions are made for maternity and maternity-related services?

11. What channels of information are routinely used for educating mothers and mothers-to-be about maternity-related services, rights, and privileges?

… peuvent être commandées, soit directement, soit par l'intermédiaire d'un …antes:

	…n Schaik's Bookstore (Pty) Ltd, P.O. Box 724, Church Street 268, PRETORIA 0001.
	Société Nationale d'Edition et de Diffusion, 3 bd Zirout Youcef, ALGER.
…D'	Govi-Verlag GmbH, Ginnheimerstrasse 20, Postfach 5360, 6236 ESCHBORN — W. E. Saarbach, Postfach 101 610, Follerstrasse 2, 5000 COLOGNE 1 — Alex. Horn, Spiegelgasse 9, Postfach 3340, 6200 WIESBADEN.
…E	Carlos Hirsch SRL, Florida 165, Galerías Güemes, Escritorio 453/465, BUENOS AIRES.
…IE	*Mail Order Sales:* Australian Government Publishing Service, P.O. Box 84, CANBERRA A.C.T. 2600; *or over the counter from* Australian Government Publishing Service Bookshops *at*: 70 Alinga Street, CANBERRA CITY A.C.T. 2600; 294 Adelaide Street, BRISBANE, Queensland 4000; 347 Swanston Street, MELBOURNE VIC 3000; 309 Pitt Street, SYDNEY N.S.W. 2000; Mt Newman House, 200 St. George's Terrace, PERTH WA 6000; Industry House, 12 Pirie Street, ADELAIDE SA 5000; 156–162 Macquarie Street, HOBART TAS 7000 — Hunter Publications, 58A Gipps Street, COLLINGWOOD VIC 3066 — R. Hill & Son Ltd., 608 St. Kilda Road, MELBOURNE, VIC 3004; Lawson House, 10–12 Clark Street, CROW'S NEST, NSW 2065.
AUTRICHE	Gerold & Co., Graben 31, 1011 VIENNE I.
BANGLADESH	Coordonnateur des Programmes OMS, G.P.O. Box 250, DACCA 5 — The Association of Voluntary Agencies, P.O. Box 5045, DACCA 5.
BELGIQUE	Office international de Librairie, 30 avenue Marnix, 1050 BRUXELLES — *Abonnements à Santé du Monde seulement*: Jean de Lannoy, 202 avenue du Roi, 1060 BRUXELLES.
BIRMANIE	*voir* Inde, Bureau régional de l'OMS.
BRÉSIL	Biblioteca Regional de Medicina OMS/OPS, Unidade de Venda de Publicações, Caixa Postal 20.381, Vila Clementino, 04023 SÃO PAULO, S.P.
CANADA	*Pour toute commande hors abonnement:* Association canadienne d'Hygiène publique, 1335 Carling Avenue, Suite 210, OTTAWA, Ontario K1Z 8N8. *Abonnements: Les demandes d'abonnement, accompagnées d'un chèque au nom de la* Banque Royale du Canada, Ottawa, compte Organisation mondiale de la Santé, *doivent être envoyées à l'*Organisation mondiale de la Santé, P.O. Box 1800, Postal Station B, OTTAWA, Ont. K1P 5R5. *La correspondance concernant les abonnements doit être adressée à l'*Organisation mondiale de la Santé, Distribution et Vente, 1211 GENÈVE 27, Suisse.
CHINE	China National Publications Import Corporation, P.O. Box 88, BEIJING (PEKING).
CHYPRE	Publishers' Distributors Cyprus, 30 Democratias Ave Ayios Dhometious, P.O. Box 4165, NICOSIA.
COLOMBIE	Distrilibros Ltd., Pío Alfonso García, Carrera 4a, N°s 36–119, CARTHAGÈNE.
DANEMARK	Munksgaard Export and Subscription Service, Nørre Søgade 35, 1370 COPENHAGUE K.
ÉGYPTE	Osiris Office for Books and Reviews, 50 Kasr El Nil Street, LE CAIRE.
EL SALVADOR	Librería Estudiantil, Edificio Comercial B Nº 3, Avenida Libertad, SAN SALVADOR.
ÉQUATEUR	Librería Científica S.A., P.O. Box 362, Luque 223, GUAYAQUIL.
ESPAGNE	Comercial Atheneum S.A., Consejo de Ciento 130–136, BARCELONE 15; General Moscardó 29, MADRID 20 — Librería Díaz de Santos, Lagasca 95 y Maldonado 6, MADRID 6; Balmes 417 y 419, BARCELONE 22.
ÉTATS-UNIS D'AMÉRIQUE	*Pour toute commande hors abonnement:* WHO Publications Centre USA, 49 Sheridan Avenue, ALBANY, N.Y. 12210. *Abonnements: Les demandes d'abonnement, accompagnées d'un chèque au nom de* Chemical Bank, New York, Account World Health Organization, *doivent être envoyées à* World Health Organization, P.O. Box 5284, Church Street Station, NEW YORK, N.Y. 10249. *La correspondance concernant les abonnements doit être adressée à l'*Organisation mondiale de la Santé, Distribution et Vente, 1211 GENÈVE 27, Suisse. *Les publications sont également disponibles auprès de* United Nations Bookshop, NEW YORK, N.Y. 10017 *(vente au détail seulement)*.
FIDJI	Coordonnateur des Programmes OMS, P.O. Box 113, SUVA.
FINLANDE	Akateeminen Kirjakauppa, Keskuskatu 2, 00101 HELSINKI 10.
FRANCE	Librairie Arnette, 2, rue Casimir-Delavigne, 75006 PARIS.
GHANA	Fides Enterprises, P.O. Box 1628, ACCRA.
GRÈCE	G. C. Eleftheroudakis S.A., Librairie internationale, rue Nikis 4, ATHÈNES (T. 126).
HAÏTI	Max Bouchereau, Librairie «A la Caravelle», Boîte postale 111-B, PORT-AU-PRINCE.
HONG KONG	Hong Kong Government Information Services, Beaconsfield House, 6th Floor, Queen's Road, Central, VICTORIA.
HONGRIE	Kultura, P.O.B. 149, BUDAPEST 62 — Akadémiai Könyvesbolt, Váci utca 22, BUDAPEST V.
INDE	Bureau régional de l'OMS pour l'Asie du Sud-Est, World Health House, Indraprastha Estate, Ring Road, NEW DELHI 110002 — Oxford Book & Stationery Co., Scindia House, NEW DELHI 110001; 17 Park Street, CALCUTTA 700016 (*Sous-agent*).
INDONÉSIE	M/s Kalman Book Service Ltd., Kwitang Raya No. 11, P.O. Box 3105/Jkt, DJAKARTA.
IRAN	Iranian Amalgamated Distribution Agency, 151 Khiaban Soraya, TÉHÉRAN.
IRAQ	Ministry of Information, National House for Publishing, Distributing and Advertising, BAGDAD.
IRLANDE	The Stationery Office, DUBLIN 4.
ISLANDE	Snaebjørn Jonsson & Co., P.O. Box 1131, Hafnarstraeti 9, REYKJAVIK.
ISRAËL	Heiliger & Co., 3 Nathan Strauss Street, JÉRUSALEM.
ITALIE	Edizioni Minerva Medica, Corso Bramante 83–85, 10126 TURIN; Via Lamarmora 3, 20100 MILAN.
JAPON	Maruzen Co. Ltd., P.O. Box 5050, TOKYO International, 100–31.
KOWEÏT	The Kuwait Bookshops Co. Ltd., Thunayan Al-Ghanem Bldg, P.O. Box 2942, KOWEÏT.
LIBAN	The Levant Distributors Co. S.A.R.L., Box 1181, Makdassi Street, Hanna Bldg, BEYROUTH.
LUXEMBOURG	Librairie du Centre, 49 bd Royal, LUXEMBOURG.

Les publications de l'OMS peuvent être commandées, soit directement, soit par l'intermédiai[re d'un] libraire, aux adresses suivantes:

MALAISIE	Coordonnateur des Programmes OMS, Room 1004, Fitzpatrick Building, Jalan Raja Chulan, K[uala] Lumpur 05–02 — Jubilee (Book) Store Ltd, 97 Jalan Tuanku Abdul Rhaman, P.O. Box 629, Ku[ala] Lumpur 01–08 — Parry's Book Center, K. L. Hilton Hotel, Jln. Treacher, P.O. Box 960, Kuala Lump[ur]
MALAWI	Malawi Book Service, P.O. Box 30044, Chichiti, Blantyre 3.
MAROC	Editions La Porte, 281 avenue Mohammed V, Rabat.
MEXIQUE	La Prensa Médica Mexicana, Ediciones Científicas, Paseo de las Facultades 26, Apt. Postal 20–413, Mexico 20, D.F.
MONGOLIE	*voir* Inde, Bureau régional de l'OMS.
MOZAMBIQUE	INLD, Caixa Postal 4030, Maputo.
NÉPAL	*voir* Inde, Bureau régional de l'OMS.
NIGÉRIA	University Bookshop Nigeria Ltd, University of Ibadan, Ibadan.
NORVÈGE	J. G. Tanum, A/S, P.O. Box 1177 Sentrum, Oslo 1.
NOUVELLE-ZÉLANDE	Government Printing Office, Publications Section, Mulgrave Street, Private Bag, Wellington 1; Walter Street, Wellington; World Trade Building, Cubacade, Cuba Street, Wellington. *Government Bookshops at:* Hannaford Burton Building, Rutland Street, Private Bag, Auckland; 159 Hereford Street, Private Bag, Christchurch; Alexandra Street, P.O. Box 857, Hamilton; T & G Building, Princes Street, P.O. Box 1104, Dunedin — R. Hill & Son Ltd, Ideal House, Cnr Gillies Avenue & Eden Street, Newmarket, Auckland 1.
PAKISTAN	Mirza Book Agency, 65 Shahrah-E-Quaid-E-Azam, P.O. Box 729, Lahore 3.
PAPOUASIE-NOUVELLE-GUINÉE	Coordonnateur des Programmes OMS, P.O. Box 5896, Boroko.
PAYS-BAS	Medical Books Europe BV, Noorderwal 38, 7241 BL Lochem.
PHILIPPINES	Bureau régional de l'OMS pour le Pacifique occidental, P.O. Box 2932, Manille — The Modern Book Company Inc., P.O. Box 632, 922 Rizal Avenue, Manille 2800.
POLOGNE	Składnica Księgarska, ul Mazowiecka 9, 00052 Varsovie *(sauf périodiques)* — BKWZ Ruch, ul Wronia 23, 00840 Varsovie *(périodiques seulement)*.
PORTUGAL	Livraria Rodriguez, 186 Rua do Ouro, Lisbonne 2.
RÉPUBLIQUE ARABE SYRIENNE	M. Farras Kekhia, P.O. Box No. 5221, Alep.
RÉPUBLIQUE DE CORÉE	Coordonnateur des Programmes OMS, Central P.O. Box 540, Séoul.
RÉPUBLIQUE DÉMOCRATIQUE ALLEMANDE	Buchhaus Leipzig, Postfach 140, 701 Leipzig.
RÉPUBLIQUE DÉMOCRATIQUE POPULAIRE LAO	Coordonnateur des Programmes OMS, P.O. Box 343, Vientiane.
ROYAUME-UNI	H.M. Stationery Office: 49 High Holborn, Londres WC1V 6HB; 13a Castle Street, Edimbourg EH2 3AR; 41 The Hayes, Cardiff CF1 1JW; 80 Chichester Street, Belfast BT1 4JY; Brazennose Street, Manchester M60 8AS; 258 Broad Street, Birmingham B1 2HE; Southey House, Wine Street, Bristol BS1 2BQ. *Toutes les commandes postales doivent être adressées de la façon suivante:* P.O. Box 569, Londres SE1 9NH.
SIERRA LEONE	Njala University College Bookshop (University of Sierra Leone), Private Mail Bag, Freetown.
SINGAPOUR	Coordonnateur des Programmes OMS, 144 Moulmein Road, G.P.O. Box 3457, Singapour 1 — Select Books (Pte) Ltd, 215 Tanglin Shopping Centre, 2/F, 19 Tanglin Road, Singapour 10.
SRI LANKA	*voir* Inde, Bureau régional de l'OMS.
SUÈDE	Aktiebolaget C.E. Fritzes Kungl. Hovbokhandel, Regeringsgatan 12, 103 27 Stockholm.
SUISSE	Medizinischer Verlag Hans Huber, Länggass Strasse 76, 3012 Berne 9.
TCHÉCOSLOVAQUIE	Artia, Ve Smeckach 30, 111 27 Prague 1.
THAÏLANDE	*voir* Inde, Bureau régional de l'OMS.
TUNISIE	Société Tunisienne de Diffusion, 5 avenue de Carthage, Tunis.
TURQUIE	Haset Kitapevi, 469 Istiklal Caddesi, Beyoglu, Istanbul.
URSS	*Pour les lecteurs d'URSS qui désirent les éditions russes:* Komsomolskij prospect 18, Medicinskaja Kniga, Moscou — *Pour les lecteurs hors d'URSS qui désirent les éditions russes:* Kuzneckij most 18, Meždunarodnaja Kniga, Moscou G-200.
VENEZUELA	Editorial Interamericana de Venezuela C.A., Apartado 50.785, Caracas 105 — Libreria del Este, Aptdo 60.337, Caracas 106 — Libreria Médica Paris, Apartado 60.681, Caracas 106.
YOUGOSLAVIE	Jugoslovenska Knjiga, Terazije 27/II, 11000 Belgrade.
ZAÏRE	Librairie universitaire, avenue de la Paix N° 167, B.P. 1682, Kinshasa I.

Des conditions spéciales sont consenties pour les pays en développement sur demande adressée aux Coordonnateurs des Programmes OMS ou aux Bureaux régionaux de l'OMS énumérés ci-dessus ou bien à l'Organisation mondiale de la Santé, Service de Distribution et de Vente, 1211 Genève 27, Suisse. Dans les pays où un dépositaire n'a pas encore été désigné, les commandes peuvent être adressées également à Genève, mais le paiement doit alors être effectué en francs suisses, en livres sterling ou en dollars des Etats-Unis.

Prix: Fr. s. 24.—

Prix sujets à modification sans préavis.